YOUR QUESTIONS ANSWERED

KT-146-930

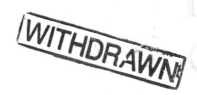

WITHDRAWN

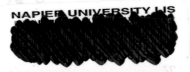

Commissioning Editor: Ellen Green
Project Development Manager: Fiona Conn, Isobel Black
Project Manager: Frances Affleck
Design Direction: George Ajayi

COPD

YOUR QUESTIONS ANSWERED

David MG Halpin
MA DPhil (OXON) MB BS (LOND) FRCP
Consultant Physician and Senior Lecturer in Respiratory Medicine
Royal Devon and Exeter Hospital, Exeter, UK

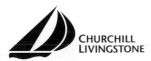

CHURCHILL
LIVINGSTONE

EDINBURGH LONDON NEW YORK OXFORD PHILADELPHIA ST LOUIS SYDNEY TORONTO 2003

CHURCHILL LIVINGSTONE
An imprint of Elsevier Science Limited

First published 2003

ISBN 0 433 07438 0

British Library Cataloguing in Publication Data
A catalogue record for this book is available from the British Library

Library of Congress Cataloging in Publication Data
A catalog record for this book is available from the Library of Congress

Notice
Medical knowledge is constantly changing. Standard safety precautions must be followed,
but as new research and clinical experience broaden our knowledge, changes in treatment
and drug therapy may become necessary or appropriate. Readers are advised to check the
most current product information provided by the manufacturer of each drug to be
administered to verify the recommended dose, the method and duration of administration,
and contraindications. It is the responsibility of the practitioner, relying on experience and
knowledge of the patient, to determine dosages and the best treatment for each individual
patient. Neither the Publisher nor the author assumes any liability for any injury and/or
damage to persons or property arising from this publication.

 ELSEVIER SCIENCE
your source for books,
journals and multimedia
in the health sciences
www.elsevierhealth.com

The
publisher's
policy is to use
**paper manufactured
from sustainable forests**

Printed in China

Contents

Preface

Nearly 1 in 10 people over 45 have COPD. It is the fifth commonest cause of death in the UK and accounts for approximately 1 million bed days per year in England alone. Despite this, many doctors believe that there is little that can be done for patients and nihilism has been rife. In the past this may have been justified, but we are entering an era when new pharmacological treatments offer considerable benefits to patients. There have also been significant advances in our understanding of the physiological benefits of these treatments and the outcome measures required to assess their effects.

Non-pharmacological therapies such as pulmonary rehabilitation and non-invasive ventilation are becoming part of routine practice and there have been important changes in the delivery of care such as hospital at-home, or assisted discharge schemes.

This book aims to provide succinct answers to questions about the role of these treatments for GPs. It also aims to answer questions about epidemiology, diagnosis and management of COPD. As well as being relevant to GPs it may be of use to specialists in training. The format allows information to be provided in an easily accessible manner and I hope it contains some information that is difficult to find elsewhere (e.g. on prognosis).

The book is organized into 14 chapters which deal with definitions and epidemiology, pathology and pathophysiology, prevention of COPD, prognosis, pharmacological management of stable disease and exacerbations, and non-pharmacological therapies. It also deals with aspects of practice organization.

Information for patients and carers is also provided at the end of each chapter and sources of further information are listed in Chapter 14.

DMGH

ACKNOWLEDGEMENTS
I would like to thank all my colleagues in primary and secondary care for their contributions to the many thought provoking discussions I have had about COPD. Writing this book would not have been possible without the understanding, support and love of Helen, Pip and Issy, to whom this book is dedicated.

How to use this book

The *Your Questions Answered* series aims to meet the information needs of GPs and other primary care professionals who care for patients with chronic conditions. It is designed to help them work with patients and their families, providing effective, evidence-based care and management.

The books are in an accessible question and answer format, with detailed contents lists at the beginning of every chapter and a complete index to help find specific information.

ICONS
Icons are used in the book to identify particular types of information:

 highlights information important to clinical practice

 highlights side effect information.

PATIENT QUESTIONS
At the end of relevant chapters there are sections of frequently asked patient questions, with easy-to-understand answers aimed at the non-medical reader. These questions are also listed at the end of the book.

Definition and epidemiology

1.1 What is COPD?

Chronic obstructive pulmonary disease (COPD) is a chronic, progressive, usually fatal disease characterized by largely irreversible obstruction of the airways that leads to breathlessness, cough, sputum production, wheeze and frequent exacerbations. It affects the airways, the alveoli, and the pulmonary vasculature and also has effects outside the lung on skeletal muscle and other organs. It is a heterogeneous disease that affects different patients in different ways.

COPD is now the recommended name for a group of conditions previously known as chronic airflow limitation (CAL), chronic obstructive airways disease (COAD), chronic obstructive lung disease (COLD), chronic bronchitis and emphysema.[1] The term was coined in the early 1960s and is preferred because it encapsulates the fact that the condition not only affects the airways but also affects the lung parenchyma and the pulmonary circulation. Recent definitions have also emphasized the inflammatory nature of the disease and the fact that it is almost always caused by inhaling tobacco smoke. Several definitions of COPD have been published, including those by the British Thoracic Society (BTS) and the Global Initiative for Obstructive Lung Disease (GOLD) (*Box 1.1*) (*see also Ch. 14*).

1.2 How is COPD related to emphysema and chronic bronchitis?

Chronic bronchitis and emphysema are specific conditions with distinct clinical or pathological features but they usually form part of the spectrum of COPD. There may also be some overlap with asthma, which if longstanding and poorly treated can lead to irreversible airflow limitation.

BOX 1.1 Definitions of COPD

- **British Thoracic Society:**[1] A chronic, slowly progressive disorder characterized by airflow obstruction (reduced forced expiratory volume in 1 second [FEV_1] and FEV_1/vital capacity [VC] ratio) that does not change markedly over several months. Most of the lung function impairment is fixed, although some reversibility can be produced by a bronchodilator (or other therapy).
- **Global Initiative for Obstructive Lung Disease:**[2] COPD is a disease state characterized by airflow limitation that is not fully reversible. The airflow limitation is usually both progressive and associated with an abnormal inflammatory response of the lungs to noxious particles or gases.

1.3　What is the difference between COPD and asthma?

COPD may develop in asthmatics who smoke and the two conditions may coexist. Some patients with COPD have partially reversible airflow limitation (*Fig. 1.1*) and this is often referred to as an 'asthmatic component'. The clinical history will usually suggest a diagnosis of asthma or COPD. The variability of airflow limitation is not dichotomous. In practice there is a spectrum of reversibility and the degree of reversibility in individual patients may vary from day to day.

There are differences in the profile of inflammatory cells present in the airways of patients with asthma and COPD but these are not amenable to routine clinical measurement.

Despite the similarities, there are important differences in the prognosis of COPD and asthma and in their respective management strategies; thus it is essential to make an accurate diagnosis.

1.4　How important is smoking as a cause of COPD?

The aetiology of COPD is multifactorial but in Western countries, cigarette smoking is unquestionably the major cause. It accounts for approximately 80% of the attributable risk.[3] There is a clear dose–response relationship between total tobacco consumption and the risk of developing COPD as well as the severity of the disease; however, not all smokers will develop COPD and susceptibility factors, possibly genetic, are also important.

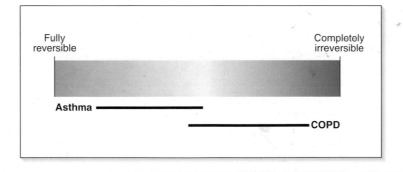

Fig. 1.1 The spectrum of reversibility of airflow obstruction in COPD and asthma.

1.5   What are the other causes of COPD?

Environmental factors and occupational dust exposures, particularly in coal miners,[4] are still important in some cases. Occupational dust exposures can cause cough and sputum production, which could be considered as bronchitis; however many of these patients do not have significant airflow obstruction and there is no loss of elastic recoil or evidence of emphysema. These patients do not, therefore, have COPD. Some occupational exposures are, however, associated with the development of COPD. The most well characterized are: cotton dust; grain dust; cement dust; oil fumes; and cadmium fumes.[5,6]

The incidence of COPD has always had a strong socioeconomic bias and this persisted even in the years when cigarette smoking was relatively evenly distributed across socio-economic groups. Low birthweight and frequent childhood infections have been associated with an increased risk of COPD[7,8] and this may partly explain the link with low socio-economic status. Similarly, damp housing and a diet low in fish, fruit and vegetables containing anti-oxidants are associated with an increased risk of COPD[9,10] and these may also explain the link with poor socio-economic status.

We do not yet know whether maternal smoking increases the risk of COPD in later life in offspring. Since it is known that maternal smoking leads to smaller airways it seems possible that it may increase the risk in children who go on to smoke.

Two other risk factors have been proposed: recurrent bronchopulmonary infections (the so-called 'British hypothesis') and pre-existing atopy and airway hyper-responsiveness (the so-called 'Dutch hypothesis').[11] There is evidence to support a role for each of these. Risk factors for COPD are summarized in *Box 1.2*.

BOX 1.2 Risk factors for COPD

- Cigarette smoking
- Age
- Dusty occupation
- Environmental pollution
- α-1 Antitrypsin deficiency
- Low birthweight
- Frequent childhood infections
- Damp housing
- Diet low in dark fish, fruit and antioxidants

1.6   How does smoking affect the lungs?

In 1976 Fletcher and colleagues published their landmark study of the natural history of airflow obstruction in COPD.[12] The key features were the more rapid loss of lung function in a proportion of smokers, the wide differences in susceptibility to developing obstruction between smokers, and the effects of quitting smoking in slowing the annual decline in FEV_1. The airflow limitation due to smoking developed gradually, even in susceptible individuals, and patients had airflow limitation for many years before becoming symptomatic.

It is now known that chronic exposure to tobacco smoke leads to an influx of inflammatory cells in to the lungs.[13] Tobacco smoke contains over 4000 chemicals, many of which are potentially toxic,[14] but it is thought that the oxidants it contains, combined with the oxidant burden from the reactive oxidant species released from the inflammatory cells it recruits are a major factor in causing COPD.[15,16] Tobacco smoke leads to the release of proteases and elastases from neutrophils and macrophages and may inhibit protective antiprotease mechanisms.[17 19] Oxidants in tobacco smoke stimulate alveolar macrophages to release pro-inflammatory mediators, some of which are chemokines. These amplify the process by recruiting other inflammatory cells to the airways; nicotine itself is also a chemotactic factor for neutrophils.[20]

1.7   Are genetic factors important?

Differences in cigarette smoking (e.g. number of cigarettes smoked in a day, number of years the person has been smoking) only account for around 15% of the variation in lung function[21] but it is still not known which factors influence an individual smoker's susceptibility to developing airflow obstruction. Family[22] and twin[23] studies have shown that genetic factors are important in COPD, but the effects are complex.[24] Extensive studies are underway to try to identify genetic risk factors.[25]

1.8   What is alpha-1 antitrypsin deficiency?

Alpha-1 antitrypsin (α-1 AT) deficiency is the only known genetic risk factor for COPD, accounting for only about 2% of cases of severe COPD.

Alpha-1 antitrypsin (or α-1 antiprotease) is the major protease inhibitor in serum and in the lung. It protects tissues against enzymatic digestion by several enzymes released by activated neutrophils, including neutrophil elastase.[26] In 1963 α-1 antitrypsin deficiency was first identified and was recognized to be associated with the early onset of severe lower zone emphysema.[27]

There is considerable variability in the clinical manifestations of patients with α-1 antitrypsin deficiency with some patients having minimal or no symptoms and others developing severe emphysema at an early age. Smoking is the major factor influencing the development of emphysema but some non-smokers develop airflow limitation in later life which appears to be associated with a history of asthma or pneumonia[28] (*see Ch. 14*).

1.9   Does the genotype matter in alpha-1 antitrypsin deficiency?

The two common forms of α-1 antitrypsin deficiency result from point mutations in the gene that codes for α-1 antitrypsin. These are known as S and Z based on the electrophoretic mobility of the protein they produce. The normal allele is known as M. The ZZ genotype results in α-1 antitrypsin levels around 10% of normal. MZ heterozygotes and SS homozygotes both have levels around 55% of normal, with MS heterozygotes having levels around 75% of normal. The SZ genotype is associated with α-1 antitrypsin levels around 40% of normal.[29] The development of emphysema is associated with deficiency of the ZZ phenotype[30] and severe deficiency of the SZ phenotype,[31] as well as with the rarer null phenotypes.[32] However, not all patients with the ZZ genotype develop emphysema, even if they are smokers.[33]

1.10   What is the British hypothesis?

The British hypothesis proposed that the decline in lung function in COPD was due to damage caused by recurrent infection.[12] Early studies could not show such an effect in relatively healthy smokers;[34,35] however, it is now clear that once airflow obstruction has developed, mucus hypersecretion and/or infections may lead to further accelerated decline in lung function.[36–39] Recent work has also shown that the lung function in patients with established COPD having frequent exacerbations often does not recover to the pre-exacerbation level before the next exacerbation occurs (*see Q. 7.4*), leading to progressive decline.

1.11   What is the Dutch hypothesis?

The Dutch hypothesis proposed that lung function declined more rapidly in smokers who had underlying airway hyper-reactivity, as is seen in asthma.[40] The effects of cigarette smoking on the rate of decline in FEV_1 are greater in the presence of airway hyper-responsiveness,[41] but it is still not known if this is a prerequisite for the development of COPD.

1.12   How common is COPD?

It is difficult to be sure how common COPD is in the general population. Many patients with mild disease are not diagnosed and do not consult their doctors and surveys based on questionnaires cannot identify patients with airflow limitation.

There is only one national study measuring airway function in patients aged 18–65 in the UK. Overall 10% of men and 11% of women had an abnormally low FEV_1.[42] In a primary care population in the UK the prevalence of an abnormal FEV_1 and respiratory symptoms was around 9% in those aged 45 years and older.[43]

1.13 Is COPD becoming less common?

There are no reliable data on the annual incidence of COPD, but as treatment does not change mortality, inferences can be made from mortality data. In men, age standardized mortality rates from COPD have fallen progressively over the last 30 years, but in women there has been a small but progressive increase over the last 20 years.[44]

1.14 What are the impacts of COPD?

COPD is one of the most common chronic diseases in the UK and in less than 20 years it will be one of the five leading medical burdens on society worldwide.[45] It results in frequent consultation in primary care, with consultation rates rising with age from 417 per year per 1000 patients aged 45–64 to 1032 per year per 1000 patients aged 75–84.[46] It is also a major burden on hospital services, accounting for around 10% of all medical admissions. COPD is estimated to cost the economy an estimated 27 million lost working days each year.

COPD accounts for over 30 000 deaths in England and Wales each year[47] but this may be an underestimate. Some patients will die with the disease rather than because of it and others will die of causes related to COPD, but their death may be certified as being due to these complications.[48]

PATIENT QUESTIONS

1.15 What is COPD?

COPD stands for **C**hronic **O**bstructive **P**ulmonary **D**isease which is now the internationally accepted term for a lung condition that causes narrowing of the airways and damage to the lung tissue. It leads to cough and breathlessness and is almost always caused by smoking.

1.16 What are the differences between COPD and emphysema or chronic bronchitis?

COPD is a term for a condition that includes different patterns of symptoms and varying amounts of damage and inflammation in the lung. Both emphysema, which is damage to the alveoli (or air sacs) in the lung where gas exchange occurs, and chronic bronchitis, which is inflammation in the large airways leading to cough and sputum production, are part of the range of changes seen in COPD.

1.17 What is the difference between COPD and asthma?

Both COPD and asthma are conditions associated with narrowing of the airways and airflow limitation. In asthma the narrowing varies significantly from day to day and within a day, whereas in COPD the narrowing is relatively fixed and does not vary to any significant extent. Studies have shown that the pattern of inflammation seen in the lungs involves different cell types in asthma and COPD.

1.18 How common is COPD?

It is difficult to know how common COPD really is as many patients with mild disease do not consult their doctor. The best estimates are that it affects at least 1 in 10 adults aged over 45.

1.19 What causes COPD?

The most important cause of COPD in Western countries is smoking. Some cases occur as a result of breathing in certain dusts at work, and a few are due to an inherited increased susceptibility to the effects of inhaled noxious dusts and chemicals.

1.20 Do all smokers develop COPD?

No. Between 1 in 5 and 1 in 3 will develop symptoms of COPD. More do not have symptoms, but show evidence of narrowing of the airways if tested. What determines whether people are affected or not is still not understood. The number of cigarettes smoked is important and people who start smoking early seem more likely to develop COPD. This is particularly true for women. Genetic factors also seem important.

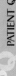

1.21   Are all forms of smoking equally bad?

COPD can be caused by smoking manufactured and self-rolled cigarettes, cigars and pipe tobacco, but there is some evidence that cigars and pipe tobacco are slightly less likely to cause COPD.

1.22   Will my children develop COPD?

Almost all cases of COPD are due to smoking but there do appear to be inherited factors which affect whether or not smokers develop COPD. If the children of a patient with COPD do not smoke they are extremely unlikely to develop COPD themselves.

1.23   What is alpha-1 antitrypsin deficiency?

Alpha-1 antitrypsin deficiency is an inherited condition which results in low levels of a protein known as alpha-1 antitrypsin. This forms part of the lung's defences against damage and patients who are deficient in alpha-1 antitrypsin are more likely to develop emphysema if they smoke (*see also Ch. 14*).

Pathology and pathophysiology

2

2.1 Does COPD just affect the airways?

As well as the changes in the airways and lung parenchyma, there are changes in the pulmonary vessels, leading to pulmonary hypertension.[49] It has also been recognized recently that COPD also affects other organs, particularly skeletal muscle, and produces systemic metabolic effects leading to weight loss.[50]

2.2 What pathological changes are seen in the airways of patients with COPD?

The airway narrowing that occurs in COPD is due to a number of causes (*Fig. 2.1*). There is narrowing and distortion of the small airways due to scarring as a consequence of the inflammation caused by smoking. There is inflammation in the peripheral airways, fibrosis in airway walls, smooth

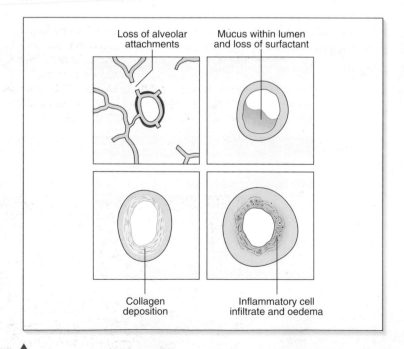

Fig. 2.1 Causes of airway obstruction.

muscle hypertrophy, goblet cell hyperplasia, mucus hypersecretion and loss of alveolar attachments which act like guy ropes to prevent the airways collapsing.[51] There are also metaplastic changes in the airway mucosa and an increase in anthracotic pigment.[52]

2.3   Which inflammatory cells are involved in COPD?

Smoking and COPD are associated with infiltration of the airway wall by CD8[+] T-lymphocytes (*Fig. 2.2*), and macrophages and neutrophils are found in the airway lumen.[51] The number of CD8[+] cells correlates with the degree of airflow limitation.[53,54] It is thought that the neutrophils move rapidly out of capillaries, through the airway wall and into the lumen[55] and that they are the key inflammatory cells. Eosinophils are not present in the airway of patients with COPD but they do appear during exacerbations.[56] Although characteristic of COPD, some of the changes in the airways can be seen in smokers who do not have airflow limitation and they persist even after stopping smoking.[57,58]

2.4   What are the pathological differences between asthma and COPD?

Unlike COPD there may be relatively few pathological features in the airways of patients with stable asthma. In asthma, there may be an inflammatory cell infiltrate in the mucosa with eosinophils and lymphocytes as the predominant cell type,[59] there may be submucosal collagen deposition and there may be disruption of the epithelium. This contrasts with the changes seen in COPD described above and the predominantly neutrophilic inflammatory cell infiltrate seen in COPD (*Table 2.1*).

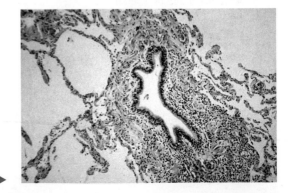

Fig. 2.2 A transverse section of a small airway in a patient with COPD showing peribronchiolitis consisting predominantly of lymphocytes. (Courtesy of Professor Peter Jeffery, Imperial College, London; *see* Jeffery.[59])

TABLE 2.1 Summary of cellular pathophysiological differences between COPD and asthma

	COPD	Asthma
Predominant cells in airways	Neutrophils	Eosinophils
Other cells present	Macrophages CD8$^+$ lymphocytes	CD4$^+$ Th2 lymphocytes Mast cells
Principal mediators	LTB4 IL-8 TNF-α	LTD4 IL-4, IL-5

2.5 What is chronic bronchitis?

Chronic bronchitis is a state of chronic mucus hypersecretion. It is associated with an increase in the volume and number of submucosal glands and the number of goblet cells in the mucosa. It was defined for the purposes of epidemiology by the British Medical Research Council as a cough productive of sputum for at least 3 months in each year for not less than 2 successive years.[60] Epidemiological studies have shown that there is no relationship between the rate of decline in the FEV$_1$ or mortality and the symptoms of chronic bronchitis.[61,62]

2.6 What is emphysema?

Emphysema is defined by the pathological changes that occur as 'a condition of the lung characterized by abnormal, permanent enlargement of airspaces distal to the terminal bronchiole accompanied by destruction of their walls and without obvious fibrosis'.[63] The distribution of the abnormal airspaces allows the classification of emphysema into panacinar, centriacinar and paraseptal. The pattern of emphysema has no effect on the clinical symptoms it produces. Bullae are areas of emphysema larger than 1 cm in diameter that are locally overdistended.[64]

2.7 What are the effects of COPD on the pulmonary circulation?

Pulmonary artery hypertension is the most important cardiovascular complication of COPD and it is associated with a poor prognosis.[65] The normal pulmonary circulation is a low-pressure, low-resistance system with low vasomotor tone. In hypoxaemic patients with COPD characteristic changes occur in peripheral pulmonary arteries: the intima of small arteries develops accumulations of smooth muscle; muscular arteries develop medial hypertrophy.[65] These structural changes may be more important in the development of sustained pulmonary hypertension than hypoxic vasoconstriction.[66] Pulmonary thrombosis may also develop, possibly secondary to small airway inflammation.[67]

2.8 What causes airway narrowing in COPD?

 Some 35 years ago it was shown that the site of airflow obstruction was the small peripheral airways.[68] Pathologically, however, the changes in these airways are subtle. Bronchioles and small bronchi derive some of their structural integrity from the attachment of surrounding alveolar walls that act like guy ropes to hold open the airway. In the presence of emphysema some of this support is lost and airflow limitation develops.[69] Other causes of small airway obstruction include: increased surface tension as a result of replacement of surfactant by inflammatory exudate; occlusion of the lumen by exudate; oedema and inflammation of the mucosa; and bronchoconstriction (*see Fig. 2.1*).

2.9 What functional abnormalities are seen in the lungs in COPD?

Decreased maximal expiratory flow and impaired gas exchange are fundamental to the pathophysiology of COPD. The effects of static airway obstruction are exacerbated by the loss of lung recoil due to destruction of the lung parenchyma.

The resting volume of the thorax is determined by the balance between the elastic recoil of the lungs and the chest wall. The floppier the lungs are the less force there is to balance the recoil of the chest wall and thus the resting thoracic volume is increased. This is in part responsible for hyperinflation seen in COPD and the increase in functional residual capacity (FRC).

Loss of lung recoil also means that the airways collapse earlier in expiration (i.e. at larger lung volumes), increasing the amount of air trapped in the lungs and again increasing the FRC and residual volume (RV). Decreased dynamic compliance also leads to the development of hyperinflation. Dynamic hyperinflation develops when the severity of airflow limitation is such that the duration of expiration is insufficient to allow the lungs to deflate fully prior to the next inspiration.

The increase in FRC greatly increases the work of breathing. In COPD both the force of contraction generated by the inspiratory muscles and the mechanical load against which they are required to act are abnormal.[70] The inspiratory load is increased as a result of the airway obstruction. The force of contraction is reduced as a consequence of the effect of hyperinflation altering the mechanical advantage of the muscles (both intercostal and diaphragmatic), malnutrition and, in some cases, respiratory muscle fatigue.

Inspiratory muscle dysfunction is central to the development of hypercapnia.[71]

2.10 Why are patients with COPD hypoxic?

The low arterial oxygen levels seen in COPD are predominantly due to gross regional variations in the balance between pulmonary blood flow and ventilation. This is due to a combination of vascular remodelling and destruction in areas of emphysema and subtle failures of the mechanisms that normally match perfusion to ventilation.[72]

2.11 Why do patients with COPD retain carbon dioxide?

Some patients with COPD have difficulty in excreting CO_2 as a result of inspiratory muscle fatigue, ventilation perfusion mismatch and possibly alveolar hypoventilation. Some of these patients respond to the difficulty in excreting CO_2 by increasing the frequency and depth of their breathing to maintain a normal arterial partial pressure of CO_2 ($PaCO_2$). However, some patients are unable to maintain adequate alveolar ventilation and there is an adaptive response in the control of breathing, with a reduced ventilatory response to the $PaCO_2$.[73] This leads to a rise in the $PaCO_2$ and the arterial partial pressure of oxygen (PaO_2) becomes an important factor in the control of breathing. Some, but not all, of these patients hypoventilate if given too much supplementary oxygen[74–76] and it is these patients who are at risk of CO_2 narcosis and respiratory arrest. There is a very poor relationship between ventilatory capacity (i.e. FEV_1) and the development of ventilatory failure.[77]

2.12 What limits exercise capacity in patients with COPD?

The relation between exercise capacity and lung function (as assessed by FEV_1) is poor[78] and the effects of bronchodilator therapy on exercise capacity correlate poorly with their effects on FEV_1. Conversely, significant improvements in exercise capacity are seen after pulmonary rehabilitation in the absence of any change in lung function. When patients with COPD exercise they stop because of breathlessness, leg discomfort or both.[78,79] Pathophysiologically, exercise limitation is due to abnormalities of ventilatory mechanics,[80] respiratory muscles,[81] gas exchange[82] and skeletal muscle function.[83] These abnormalities may be present even in patients with mild disease.[84]

■ Ventilatory factors are probably the most important. Expiratory flow rates in patients with COPD are close to maximal even at rest; this means that the lungs are not able to empty fully during the higher frequency of breathing during exercise, leading to increased air trapping.[85] This dynamic hyperinflation limits exercise capacity by increasing the work of breathing. The degree of dynamic hyperinflation that develops varies considerably from patient to patient.[86] Patients attempt to overcome dynamic hyperinflation by recruiting abdominal and expiratory intercostal muscles during expiration[87] but this further increases the work of breathing.[88] These effects appear to be important in patients with mild disease as well as in those with more severe disease.[89]

■ Skeletal muscle dysfunction is another important determinant of exercise tolerance[90] that explains the poor correlation with FEV_1. Peak exercise capacity is proportional to skeletal muscle mass and strength.[83,91] The causes of skeletal muscle dysfunction probably vary from patient to patient[92] and include deconditioning, malnutrition, hypoxia, hypercapnia and increased oxidative stress.

2.13 What is dynamic hyperinflation and why is it important?

Dynamic hyperinflation is the term used to describe the increase in air trapping that occurs in patients with COPD when they exercise. The expiratory flow limitation that is characteristic of COPD means that there is little scope for increasing expiratory flow rates during exercise. Thus, when the respiratory rate is increased during exercise, the lungs are not able to empty fully, leading to increased air trapping.[85] The degree of dynamic hyperinflation that develops varies considerably from patient to patient.[86]

Dynamic hyperinflation is important because it increases the work of breathing. This is because the lungs are less compliant at higher volumes and greater inspiratory loads are present due to the increased elastic recoil of the chest wall at higher volumes. In an attempt to compensate for the effects of dynamic hyperinflation, abdominal and expiratory intercostal muscles are often recruited during expiration[87] but this further increases the work of breathing.[88]

Dynamic hyperinflation contributes to the respiratory discomfort during exercise[93,94] and changes in dynamic hyperinflation produced by bronchodilator therapy or lung volume reduction surgery correlate with improvements in exercise capacity.[95,96]

PATIENT QUESTIONS

2.14 How does COPD affect the lungs?

COPD causes inflammation in the walls of the air tubes in the lungs (the bronchi). This causes scarring in the walls of these tubes and some spasm of the muscles in the walls of the air tubes, both of which lead to narrowing of the air tubes and difficulty breathing in and out. Inflammation also leads to increased production of mucus in the air tubes and this is coughed up as phlegm. COPD also causes damage to the air sacs (alveoli), which are where oxygen is absorbed into the blood stream. This damage, which is known as emphysema, leads to low oxygen levels that limit the ability to do things and also leads to breathlessness.

2.15 Does COPD just affect the lungs?

The majority of symptoms in COPD are due to its effects on the air tubes (bronchi) and air sacs (alveoli) but COPD also affects the blood vessels in the lungs and can put a strain on the heart. COPD also has some effects on other parts of the body, including the muscles in the arms and legs.

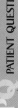

Diagnosis and prognosis

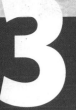

DIAGNOSIS

3.1   How is COPD diagnosed?

The diagnosis is largely made on the clinical grounds in patients who have smoked. It is confirmed by demonstrating airflow obstruction that shows little day to day or diurnal variation and minimal response to bronchodilators. Airflow obstruction can only be accurately shown by spirometry rather than by measuring peak flow rates.

■ Many patients will only present at the time of an exacerbation and will be unaware that they have a chronic illness (*see Q. 7.1*). Some will have had a cough or been breathless for some time but will not have recognized that these were symptoms of a lung condition. It is often only in retrospect that patients realize that they have been breathless on exertion or have had a productive cough for several years. Many smokers have a morning cough that they regard as normal for them and become breathless on exertion, which they regard as a part of normal ageing.

■ Age is a risk factor for COPD and the presence of symptoms suggestive of a diagnosis of COPD in patients under the age of 40 should raise the possibility of an alternative diagnosis or an unusual aetiology such as α-1 antitrypsin deficiency.

3.2   What are the symptoms of COPD?

Patients with mild airflow obstruction are often asymptomatic, but as COPD develops patients become progressively more symptomatic. The relationship of symptoms to different levels of physiological abnormality and the rate of progression can be very variable.

The cardinal symptoms of COPD are cough, wheeze and breathlessness. When patients do first develop symptoms these are usually mild and intermittent. Patients with moderate COPD invariably have some symptoms, but again the spectrum is wide. Patients with severe COPD are almost always breathless on minimal exertion, and their sleep may be disturbed by breathlessness. They generally cough, especially in the mornings, and frequently wheeze. In addition they may have symptoms of complications such as peripheral oedema.

In 75% of patients with COPD cough is one of the first symptoms, either preceding or developing simultaneously with breathlessness. It may be productive of sputum and is generally worse in the morning. In the absence of infection, the sputum may vary in colour from clear, through white to grey. Purulent (green or brown) sputum can be a sign of infection but can also simply be a reflection of the neutrophil trafficking seen as part of the inflammatory process.

Breathlessness usually develops insidiously and may be regarded as a normal part of ageing. Patients often modify their behaviour to avoid activities that provoke breathlessness and thus may not experience this symptom. Subjective breathlessness correlates poorly with the degree of airflow obstruction. It can be quantified by asking about exercise tolerance (e.g. the distance the patient can walk on the flat or the number of flights of stairs they can climb before having to stop) or by using a scale such as the

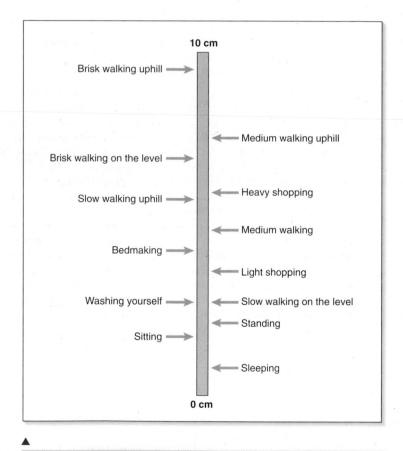

Fig. 3.1 The oxygen cost diagram. Patients mark the point on the line above which they become breathless.

TABLE 3.1	Medical Research Council dyspnoea scale
Grade	**Degree of breathlessness related to activities**
1	Not troubled by breathlessness except on strenuous exercise
2	Short of breath when hurrying or walking up a slight hill
3	Walks slower than contemporaries on the level because of breathlessness, or has to stop for breath when walking at own pace
4	Stops for breath after walking about 100 m or after a few minutes on the level
5	Too breathless to leave the house, or breathless when dressing or undressing

oxygen cost diagram (*Fig. 3.1*) or the UK's Medical Research Council (MRC) dyspnoea scale (*Table 3.1*).

Unlike asthma, the breathlessness of COPD does not vary markedly from day to day or within a day, and patients' exercise capacity is fairly constant. Breathlessness may vary according to environmental conditions and often worsens in smoky or dusty atmospheres. It is also sensitive to changes in the weather, particularly temperature and humidity. The lack of good and bad days is a useful pointer to the diagnosis of COPD.

Chest pain may be a feature of COPD and is thought to be related to intercostal muscle ischaemia, but other causes such as infection, tumours or ischaemic heart disease should be excluded.

Ankle swelling occurs as a consequence of the development of cor pulmonale. It often worsens at times of exacerbation (*see Q. 7.6*). Weight loss is a common symptom in advanced COPD. It is due to a combination of the effects of the increased work of breathing, reduced calorie intake because of increased breathlessness and the metabolic effects of COPD. However, it may also be a feature of lung cancer, and rapid weight loss (particularly if associated with other symptoms) should always be investigated.

The exercise limitation, frustration and social isolation produced by COPD often leads to clinical depression. Common symptoms in COPD are summarized in *Box 3.1*.

3.3   What are the findings on examination?

The findings on clinical examination in patients with COPD are as variable as the symptoms.

Examination is often normal in patients with asymptomatic or mild disease. In patients with moderate disease there may be signs of hyperinflation (depressed liver, loss of cardiac dullness, reduced cricosternal

---

BOX 3.1 Common symptoms in COPD

■ Breathlessness
■ Cough
■ Wheeze
■ Frequent winter 'bronchitis'
■ Chest pain
■ Ankle swelling
■ Weight loss
■ Depression

---

distance, increased anteroposterior diameter of chest). Polyphonic wheezes or abnormally quiet breath sounds may be heard. If there is a component of chronic bronchitis coarse crackles may be heard. Expiration is prolonged. There is a very poor correlation between the clinical signs and the severity of airflow obstruction.

In patients with severe disease the findings on examination may include: signs of hyperinflation (as above), wheezes, quiet breath sounds, peripheral oedema, elevated venous pressure, central cyanosis, right ventricular heave, loud pulmonary second sound, tricuspid regurgitation, signs of hypercapnia (flapping tremor, bounding pulse, drowsiness), and weight loss or cachexia. Clinical signs in COPD are summarized in *Box 3.2*.

3.4 What are pink puffers and blue bloaters?

Historically, patients have been divided into 'blue bloaters' and 'pink puffers': the latter maintain relatively normal blood gases through a drive to breathe that can be extremely distressing. The former are patients who are hypoxaemic and hypercapnic as a result of acclimatization of their

---

BOX 3.2 Clinical signs of COPD

■ None
■ Hyperinflated chest
■ Wheeze or quiet breath sounds
■ Pursed lip breathing
■ Use of accessory muscles
■ Peripheral oedema
■ Cyanosis
■ Raised jugular venous pressure (JVP)
■ Cachexia

BOX 3.3 Differential diagnosis of COPD

■ Asthma
■ Bronchiectasis
■ Left ventricular dysfunction
■ Carcinoma of the bronchus
■ Obliterative bronchiolitis

---

regulatory centres and a reduced drive to breathe. They frequently have peripheral oedema as a reflection of pulmonary hypertension and cor pulmonale. In practice these are extremes of a spectrum and most patients lie somewhere in the middle. There is no firm relationship with the predominance of airflow obstruction or emphysema.

These terms are not now widely used.

3.5 What other conditions may present with similar symptoms and signs?

The differential diagnosis of patients presenting with symptoms suggestive of COPD is shown in *Box 3.3*. The differentiation of asthma from COPD is discussed below. Some patients will have both COPD and left ventricular dysfunction, but in others the symptoms will be entirely due to another condition (e.g. bronchiectasis) and these patients may require referral for a specialist opinion.

3.6 Can early COPD be identified by screening?

Most patients have smoked at least 20 cigarettes per day for at least 20 years before they develop symptoms; however, airflow obstruction may develop sooner and is usually present for some years before symptoms develop. If airflow obstruction is detected at this stage progression to symptomatic COPD may be prevented by stopping the patient smoking. The identification of these presymptomatic individuals presents a challenge for health promotion programmes, but now that effective anti-smoking interventions are available there is a greater incentive to try to identify these patients using spirometry as a screening tool.[97]

SPIROMETRY

3.7 What is spirometry?

Spirometry measures the volume of air exhaled in 1 second (the FEV_1) and the total amount of air exhaled (the FVC) when the patient inhales maximally and then exhales as forcefully and deeply as possible. By comparing these volumes with those predicted for the patient's age, sex and

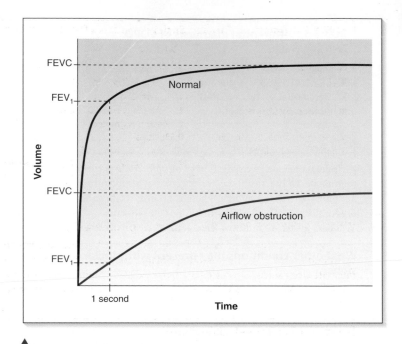

Fig. 3.2 Time/volume curves showing the FEV$_1$ and FVC in normal subjects and in patients with airflow obstruction due to, for example, COPD.

height, and computing the ratio of the FEV$_1$ to FVC it is possible to diagnose airflow obstruction with confidence (*Fig. 3.2*). It is also possible to diagnose mild airflow obstruction and to assess the severity of airflow obstruction. As well as measuring the FVC, spirometers can be used to measure the vital capacity (VC).

3.8   What are FEV$_1$, FVC, SVC and VC?

The FEV$_1$ (forced expiratory volume in 1 second) is the volume of air exhaled in 1 second when the patient inhales maximally and then exhales as forcefully and deeply as possible. The FVC (forced vital capacity) is the total volume of air exhaled during this manoeuvre. The SVC (slow vital capacity) is the volume of air exhaled in a slow, non-forced manner after a maximum inhalation. It is also known as the vital capacity (VC). The VC is often greater than the FVC in diseases such as COPD, where the airways are floppy and collapse prematurely during a forced manoeuvre.

TABLE 3.2 American Thoracic Society standards for spirometers	
Feature	**Standard**
FEV_1 and FVC range	0.5–8 litres
Accuracy	± 5% reading or ± 0.100 litres, whichever is greater
Reproducibility (precision)	± 3% reading or ± 0.050 litres, whichever is greater
Minimum detectable volume	0.030 litres
Duration of volume acquisition	At least 15 seconds
Display	Paper record or graphical display required

3.9 What are the important features of a spirometer?

Some spirometers measure exhaled volumes directly but these models are bulky and most spirometers used in primary care measure flow and integrate electronically over time to derive exhaled volumes. Spirometers should meet the American Thoracic Society (ATS) standards, as outlined in *Table 3.2*.

3.10 Do spirometers need calibrating?

Quality control in spirometry is essential if the results are to be accurate and meaningful. Spirometers need regular calibration, which is quick and easy to do. The usual method is to use a 3 litre calibration syringe with different injection times to give flow rates between 2 and 12 litres per second (i.e. taking approximately 1 second and 6 seconds to inject 3 litres).[98–101] As well as using a calibration syringe it is a good idea to have a few 'biological controls' (i.e. members of staff) who perform spirometry on a regular basis. A calibration log which records the results of the calibrations should be kept.

3.11 Do spirometers need cleaning?

Spirometers need regular cleaning and servicing. Transmission of infection is a possibility during spirometry if infection control measures are not adequate.[102] There is a possibility of transmission of upper and lower respiratory tract infections, tuberculosis and other infections via both direct contact on the mouthpiece and inhalation of contaminated aerosol droplets from fluid accumulating in the mouthpiece and tubing. To avoid such cross-contamination, mouthpieces should be disposable, tubing (if required) should be either disinfected or sterilized on a regular basis, and patients should be instructed not to inhale through the device.[103] If electronic devices are used the manufacturer's instructions regarding cleaning should be followed.

3.12 How should spirometry be performed?

For the results of spirometry to be meaningful the measurement must be made properly. Both the British Thoracic Society (BTS) with the Associated of Respiratory Technicians and Physiologists (ARTP) and the American Thoracic Society have published guidelines on the performance of spirometry.[103,104] Production of reliable results is very dependent on the person performing the test with the patient. They must understand the criteria for an adequate manoeuvre (*Box 3.4*) and must have the ability to coax the patient to perform a maximal forced exhalation. They will often need to demonstrate the manoeuvre first. Spirometry is best supervised by people who do it regularly and many practices find it convenient to concentrate the skills in one or two practice nurses.

Patients should be sitting, unless they are very obese. Exhalation should continue for at least 6 seconds and the test should not be stopped until the volume trace has reached a plateau for at least 2 seconds or the exhalation has continued for at least 15 seconds. The results of the measurement should only be accepted if the manoeuvre is performed with maximal effort and if the trace is smooth and cough free. The patient should perform at least three manoeuvres and the FVC should be within 5% in two out of the three. The best FEV_1 and the best FVC are recorded.

Common problems when performing spirometry include:

- previous inspiration was not complete (i.e. total lung capacity was not reached)
- exhalation begins before the patient connects to the mouthpiece
- a leak between the lips and the mouthpiece
- exhalation was performed through pursed lips or partially closed teeth
- exhalation was not maximally forced or sustained to residual volume
- exhalation was interrupted by coughing or premature inhalation.

BOX 3.4 Criteria for an acceptable spirometric manoeuvre

- Full inspiration
- Good seal with mouthpiece
- Maximum effort used
- No coughing
- No premature inhalation
- Exhalation continues for at least 6 seconds
- Volume trace has reached a plateau

3.13 How can I learn how to perform spirometry?

Spirometry is not difficult to perform and it is easy to learn how to do it properly. Training in the use of spirometers and interpretation of the results is widely available. The BTS COPD Consortium has produced a very popular guide to performing and interpreting spirometry entitled *Spirometry in Practice*. This is available free of charge from the Consortium and can also be downloaded from their section of the BTS web site (*www.brit-thoracic.org.uk*).

Many hospitals in the UK offer training in spirometry for their local primary care teams. Spirometry training is also provided nationally by organisations such as the National Respiratory Training Centre (NRTC) or the Respiratory Education and Training Centres (RETC) (*see Ch. 14*). For those wanting a more academic qualification, the BTS/ARTP offer a certificate in spirometry. Candidates are required to achieve a satisfactory standard in a practical examination, an oral examination and an assignment. Many manufacturers also offer instruction and advice on the correct use of their spirometer (*see Ch. 14*).

3.14 How do I interpret the results of spirometry?

The results of spirometry must be interpreted in the light of the predicted values for that patient. The reference values most commonly used in Europe are those produced by a working party of the European Respiratory Society.[105] Many spirometers now calculate the predicted values for an individual once their age, sex and height have been entered, but tables of normal values are widely available.

3.15 What is the role of spirometry?

The presence of airflow limitation is best assessed using spirometry. A normal FEV_1 effectively excludes the diagnosis of COPD but a normal peak expiratory flow rate (PEFR) does not. It has been suggested that significant day to day or diurnal peak flow variability of more than 20% indicates a large reversible component to the airflow obstruction; however, at low absolute values the spontaneous variability in PEFR may exceed this value.[106]

Uses of FEV_1 in COPD include diagnosis, assessing severity, assessing prognosis and monitoring progression.

3.16 Can peak flow rates be used in place of spirometry?

Measurement of peak expiratory flow (PEF) rates has proved extremely useful in the monitoring of patients with asthma but it frequently underestimates the severity of airflow obstruction in COPD. This is because in COPD the airways are generally floppy and the degree of airflow obstruction shows significant volume dependency. Thus, at large lung volumes the flow limitation is less severe and the *peak* expiratory flow rate is relatively well preserved; at lower lung volumes, however, the expiratory flow rate is severely limited. This is reflected in a reduction in the FEV_1.[107]

Spirometry has several other advantages over the measurement of PEF rates. It is more reproducible and low readings, due to poor technique or inadequate effort, are easily identified. The BTS COPD guidelines recommend that spirometry is available in primary care or that an open access service is provided by secondary care. There are many advantages for practices that own their own spirometer, not least the immediacy with which results are available.

3.17 Can spirometry diagnose COPD?

Airflow obstruction is fundamental to the diagnosis of COPD and this can only be accurately assessed using spirometry. Spirometry does not itself differentiate between airflow obstruction due to asthma and that due to COPD but when the results are interpreted in the context of the clinical setting it is a sensitive way of diagnosing COPD. If the diagnosis remains unclear, changes in spirometry after administration of bronchodilators or corticosteroids may help clarify this. It is also important to remember that asthma and COPD may coexist.

3.18 What is a reversibility test?

Spirometry alone cannot diagnose COPD, it will merely show the presence of airflow obstruction. Reversibility testing has been used to assess the variability of the airflow obstruction, often as a means of differentiating asthma from COPD. In practice there is a spectrum of reversibility that overlaps with asthma. Reversibility can be assessed acutely with short-acting bronchodilators or over a period of weeks with oral or inhaled corticosteroids. Responses to bronchodilators may vary from day to day and the thresholds for defining a positive response are largely arbitrary; as yet there is no agreement over the best way of defining this.[108] Volume responses of 400 ml or more are suggestive of asthma.[109]

Short-term changes in FEV_1 in response to bronchodilators or steroids do not predict long-term clinical responses[110–113] and should not be used to guide therapy.

Steroid reversibility testing (protocols for which are outlined in *Box 3.5*) may show significant improvements in FEV_1 when bronchodilator reversibility testing has not. For this reason it is often performed in preference to a bronchodilator reversibility test.

Steroid reversibility testing is not usually required in patients with mild

---

BOX 3.5 Steroid reversibility testing protocols

Spirometry before and after:

- 2 weeks of treatment with 30 mg prednisolone daily.
- 6 weeks of treatment with 800–1000 µg inhaled steroids daily.

---

disease but should be carried out in all patients with moderate and severe disease. FEV_1 should be measured before and at the end of a course of oral steroids. A positive response will usually be produced in patients treated with 30 mg prednisolone daily within 2 weeks, but some clinicians continue the trial for up to 4 weeks. Inhaled steroids can also be used, but in this case the trial should continue for 6 weeks with doses equivalent to 1000 mg beclometasone per day; a negative response may be influenced by poor compliance or inhaler technique.

The response should be assessed by measuring the pre- and post-trial FEV_1. An increase in FEV_1 of 400 ml or more is suggestive of asthma. The 1997 BTS guidelines proposed that a change in FEV_1 that was both more than 200 ml and more than 15% of the pre-test value was interpreted as significant reversibility. A rise in FEV_1 of more than 200 ml is associated with a better prognosis over the next 5 years.[114]

Some patients report a subjective improvement following steroid therapy but do not show significant objective improvements. Such patients should not be considered as having a positive response and should not continue on oral corticosteroids. Failure to respond to a steroid trial when clinically stable does not mean that patients should not receive steroids during an exacerbation because different inflammatory cells are involved at these times (*see Qs 7.13 and 7.16*).

Reversibility testing with bronchodilators gives information about prognosis but the acute response to bronchodilators in this setting has relatively little bearing on the subsequent subjective or objective response to bronchodilator therapy: a negative result does not mean that patients will not derive symptomatic benefits, in terms of perception of breathlessness and increases in walking distance, from treatment with bronchodilators.

If undertaken, reversibility testing with bronchodilators should be carried out in a way that ensures that a failure to respond is not because the dose is too low. For this reason it is best to use nebulised drugs and both beta agonists (e.g. salbutamol or terbutaline) and anticholinergics should be used either sequentially or in combination. For simplicity and to maximize the predictive value of the test it is best to use a combination of salbutamol and ipratropium delivered via a nebuliser.

Tests should be performed when patients are clinically stable and free of infection. The patient should not have taken a short acting bronchodilator

---

BOX 3.6 Bronchodilator reversibility testing protocols
- Patient must be clinically stable
- Patients should avoid:
    - short-acting β-agonist for 6 hours
    - long-acting β-agonist for 12 hours
    - sustained release theophylline for 24 hours
- Baseline spirometry
- Nebulised salbutamol (2.5 mg) and ipratropium (500 μg)
- Wait 30 minutes
- Repeat spirometry

---

in the previous 6 hours, a long acting beta agonist in the previous 12 hours or a sustained release theophylline preparation in the previous 24 hours. As with steroid trials, the response should be assessed by measuring the pre- and post-trial FEV_1. An increase in FEV_1 that is both more than 200 ml and more than 15% of the pre-test value was again the threshold recommended by the BTS for establishing reversibility, but absolute increases of 400 ml or more are probably of greater clinical significance. Bronchodilator reversibility testing protocols are summarized in *Box 3.6*.

3.19 Does reversibility testing help choose the best treatment for a patient?

Single dose bronchodilator reversibility tests are important in the assessment of patients with COPD; however, they do not predict the symptomatic benefit that patients may obtain from bronchodilator therapy.[111] Bronchodilators may increase FEV_1, FVC or exercise tolerance independently, but an increase in FEV_1 does not correlate well with an improvement in symptoms. As well as increasing airway calibre, these drugs lead to a reduction in pulmonary hyperinflation, increase mucociliary clearance, and improve respiratory muscle function.[115] All of these actions may contribute to the clinical benefit but most trials have only used changes in FEV_1 as the outcome measure.

3.20 How can the severity of COPD be assessed using spirometry?

The BTS guidelines propose a classification of COPD into mild, moderate and severe based on FEV_1. Patients' health needs are related to these categories, and exacerbation rates (*see Q. 7.5*) and the risk of hospitalization increase as the FEV_1 falls.

Guidelines on the management of COPD, containing recommendations on severity assessment, have also been published by the American Thoracic Society (ATS), the European Respiratory Society (ERS) and most recently by the Global Initiative for Chronic Obstructive Lung Disease (GOLD)[116–118] (*see also Ch. 14*). All four define severity in slightly different ways. The BTS guidelines use FEV_1 (as a percentage of the predicted) to define severity with three bands: 60–80%, 40–60% and less than 40% to define mild, moderate and severe COPD. The GOLD guidelines recommended definitions based mainly on the FEV_1, but also take account of the presence of heart failure and include an 'at risk' stage. New ATS/ERS guidelines currently in development suggest new thresholds of 50–80%, 30–50% and less than 30% predicted.

3.21 Where can I get spirometry performed if I don't have a spirometer in my practice?

Many hospitals now run open access spirometry clinics which can provide measurements on patients referred from primary care. There has also been interest in providing spirometry services at a primary care trust level.[119]

OTHER TESTS

3.22 What other lung function tests may be useful in diagnosing COPD?

Laboratory lung function tests measuring static lung volumes, i.e. total lung capacity (TLC), residual volume (RV) and functional residual capacity (FRC), and gas transfer are useful in some patients, particularly those in whom the level of breathlessness or functional impairment appears disproportionate to the degree of airflow limitation measured by spirometry.

3.23 What other tests should be performed?

The ECG is useful for detecting ischaemic heart disease and arrhythmias but is relatively insensitive for detecting right ventricular hypertrophy. ECG criteria for ventricular hypertrophy are modified by hyperinflation of the lungs.

Echocardiography is a useful way of identifying right ventricular hypertrophy and dilatation; however, hyperinflation increases the retrosternal air space thus making satisfactory transthoracic studies difficult. Where available, transoesophageal echocardiography increases the proportion of satisfactory examinations. Pulmonary artery (PA) pressure can be estimated using echocardiography in a number of ways. The blood velocity in the main PA can be used to estimate the PA pressure and the interval between the onset of right ventricular (RV) ejection and peak velocity correlates well with the mean PA pressure. In patients with tricuspid regurgitation, the addition of the mean right atrial (RA) pressure to the peak systolic gradient between the RA and RV yields the systolic PA pressure.

Identification of anaemia and polycythaemia is useful in the management of patients with COPD. Patients with a haematocrit > 47% in women or > 52% in men should be investigated for hypoxaemia, including at night. Venesection should be considered if the packed cell volume (PCV) is greater than 60% in men or 55% in women; however, the evidence for its benefits in terms of improved exercise performance and reduced risk of vascular events is limited, as is evidence regarding the duration of benefit.

3.24 Is sputum culture helpful?

Routine sputum culture is of no value in the management of patients with stable COPD. Sputum is frequently colonized with bacteria such as *Haemophilus influenzae* whose identification, in itself, is not an indication for antibiotic therapy.

During an acute exacerbation sputum usually becomes purulent (*see Qs 7.6 and 7.15*) and this is one of the defining features. A Gram stain may show a mixture of organisms, similar to those cultured when the patient is stable. These may include *Streptococcus pneumoniae*, *H. influenzae* and *Moraxella catarrhalis*. If thought appropriate, antibiotic therapy is usually started before the results of sputum culture are available, but occasionally has to be modified on the basis of culture results and lack of response to empirical therapy.

3.25 Is a chest X-ray necessary to diagnose COPD?

The plain chest radiograph is frequently unremarkable in patients with stable mild disease. As such it contributes little to the diagnosis but its role lies in excluding other diagnoses such as a bronchogenic carcinoma (*Fig. 3.3*). It may show hyperinflation, bronchial wall thickening, a paucity of vascular markings or single or multiple bullae, but may be surprisingly normal in patients with significant emphysema as assessed by gas transfer measurements or by computed tomography (CT). All patients with COPD should have a chest radiograph at the time of diagnosis to exclude these other conditions and should have further radiographs if they develop any worrying symptoms such as haemoptysis or are slow to recover from an exacerbation.

In patients with exacerbations, plain chest radiographs are again principally useful for excluding other causes of the patient's symptoms such as lobar pneumonia or pneumothorax (*see Qs 7.8 and 7.15*).

3.26 What is the role of CT scanning in diagnosing COPD?

CT is good at showing the presence of emphysema but is only rarely clinically indicated for this purpose. Examples of its use are as part of a

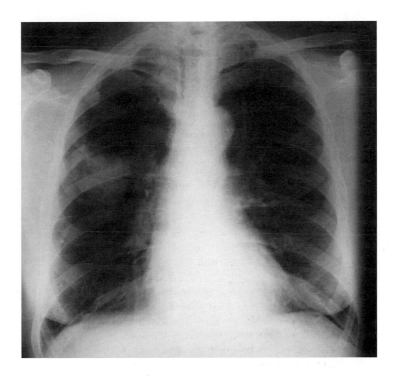

▲
Fig. 3.3 A chest radiograph showing a right mid zone carcinoma in a woman with COPD.

work-up for bullectomy, lung volume reduction surgery or single lung transplantation, and to confirm the presence of emphysema in young patients with isolated low gas transfer measurements (e.g. α1-antitrypsin deficiency).

3.27 What is pulse oximetry?

Pulse oximetry can be used to assess hypoxaemia at rest and on exertion in patients with stable disease and during exacerbations. If the SaO_2 is more than 92% in patients with stable disease, measurement of arterial blood gas tensions is probably not required. If the SaO_2 is < 92% arterial blood gas tensions should be measured and measurement of arterial blood gases should be considered in all patients with an exacerbation (*see Qs 7.15 and 7.16*) as their $PaCO_2$ may be abnormal even if their SaO_2 is normal.

3.28 How does pulse oximetry help in the management of COPD?

Pulse oximetry can be used to identify patients who may need long term oxygen therapy. It can also help guide patients about whether they need oxygen during air travel and can be used as part of the assessment of patients with exacerbations of COPD to identify those patients who need admitting to hospital (*see Qs 7.9 and 7.16*).

3.29 How can patients with COPD be differentiated from those with asthma?

In most cases, the history, examination and investigations will enable patients with asthma to be distinguished from those with COPD (*Table 3.3*). Particular pointers are the age of the patient, their smoking history and evidence of variability in airflow obstruction (either serial PEF or reversibility testing). This distinction is important and attempts should be made accurately to classify all patients.

3.30 How can exercise capacity be assessed in patients with COPD?

Exercise capacity in COPD can be assessed in a variety of ways ranging from full cardiopulmonary exercise testing in a lung function laboratory to self-assessment of walking distance. Three basic types of exercise test can be performed: progressive symptom limited tests, steady state exercise tests and self-paced exercise tests. Each gives slightly different information and can be performed using a variety of methods.

Formal cardiopulmonary exercise testing gives extensive information about ventilatory, cardiovascular and metabolic performance during

TABLE 3.3 Pointers that differentiate asthma from COPD		
	COPD	Asthma
History		
Smoker or ex-smoker	Nearly all	Possibly
Symptoms under age 45	Uncommon	Often
Chronic *productive* cough	Common	Uncommon
Breathlessness	Persistent and progressive	Variable
Winter bronchitis	Common	Uncommon
Investigations		
Spirometry	Obstructive picture	May be normal
Serial peak expiratory flow	Minimal variation	Day to day and diurnal variation
Reversibility testing	Variable	Often > 400 ml change

exercise but it is often difficult for patients to undertake and is largely a research tool.[120]

Timed walking tests, particularly the 6 minute walking test,[121,122] can be used to assess exercise capacity but it has been shown that changes of at least 54 m in the overall distance walked are required for the average patient to notice a difference in their functional status.[123] Timed walking tests are also susceptible to factors that influence motivation[124] and for this reason a timed incremental shuttle walk has been developed.[125] The test consists of a flat course with cones 10 m apart. A cassette tape gives standardized instructions to the patient and controls the progress of the test with a series of beeps. The walking speed increases over stages lasting 1 minute and the test ends when the patient fails to reach the cone in the designated time period or becomes too breathless to continue. These tests are still potentially influenced by familiarity and several walks on different days may be required before a plateau is reached.

Incremental exercise testing measures different parameters from endurance testing where patients perform submaximal exercise for as long as possible. Most activities of daily living are performed at submaximal exercise levels and thus endurance tests may relate better to patients' functional status. An endurance shuttle walking test based on the incremental test has also been developed.[126] This is simple to perform, has good repeatability over time and is sensitive to changes produced by pulmonary rehabilitation.

All walking tests suffer from the fact that patients with mild or moderate COPD are not sufficiently stressed to reach their maximum exercise capacity.

PROGNOSIS AND NATURAL HISTORY

3.31 What is the natural history of COPD?

The best information on the natural history of airflow obstruction in COPD is still the pioneering study of Fletcher and colleagues.[127] The key findings were that COPD developed in a proportion of smokers who experienced a more rapid loss of lung function as a result of smoking. There were wide differences in susceptibility to developing obstruction between smokers and in the effects of quitting smoking on slowing the annual decline in FEV_1. The airflow limitation due to smoking developed gradually, even in susceptible individuals, and patients had airflow limitation for many years before becoming symptomatic. Similar findings were reported by Burrows in the USA.[128]

The Lung Health Study has shown that the accelerated loss of lung function in smokers continues in patients with mild to moderate COPD. Stopping smoking returns the rate of loss of lung function to the value seen in non-smokers.[129]

The loss of lung function in susceptible smokers may remain asymptomatic for many years.[130] Functional impairment and disability often appear to develop fairly rapidly in patients in their late forties and fifties when the pulmonary reserve has been exhausted. Vestbo and Lange showed that 4.9% of over 6200 smokers who did not have airflow obstruction went on to develop mild COPD within 5 years and 6.7% went on to develop moderate COPD.[131] The presence of symptoms, for example cough and sputum in the absence of airflow obstruction (i.e. GOLD stage zero), did not increase the risk of developing COPD.

3.32 How long do patients with COPD survive?

Even mild COPD in patients needing no treatment appears to reduce survival. Survival is worse in patients with more severe disease.[132] Most patients are not diagnosed until they are in their fifties. Five year survival from diagnosis is 78% in men and 72% in women with mild disease but falls to 30% in men and 24% in women with severe disease. The mean age of death of patients with severe COPD was 74.2 years compared with 77.2 years in patients with mild disease and 78.3 years in controls. Patients with moderate COPD had an intermediate survival with a mean age at death of 76.6 years (J.B. Soriano, personal communication).

3.33 What do COPD patients die of?

There is surprisingly little information on this. Data collected on the causes of death in patients on long term oxygen therapy showed that about one in three died of acute or chronic respiratory failure. Heart failure was the next most common cause of death (13%), followed by pulmonary infection, pulmonary embolism, cardiac arrhythmia and lung cancer. A similar picture was reported over 30 years ago,[133] although it is difficult to be sure that all these patients had COPD. Large population studies in Finland have looked at the causes of death in patients who had had a hospital admission for COPD and again found that respiratory failure, ischaemic heart disease and lung cancer were the three most common causes of death.[134,135] This has also been found in smaller studies in selected populations.[136]

3.34 What factors predict outcome in COPD?

Post-bronchodilator FEV_1 is a good indicator of prognosis in COPD.[137] Pre-bronchodilator FEV_1 is also predictive of outcome but the predictive value is slightly less good.[138] Patients with a low body mass index (BMI) also have an increased mortality[139,140] although it has recently been shown that muscle mass or lean body mass is a better predictor of outcome than total body mass.[141] Dyspnoea, as assessed by the MRC respiratory symptoms questionnaire,[142] has also been suggested as an independent predictor of outcome,[143] and as the disease is progressive, age itself is also an important predictor of outcome.[144] Recently it has been shown that poor health-related quality of life is also a poor prognostic factor.[145]

Gas transfer, as assessed by the transfer coefficient,[146–148] the PaO_2,[149] and the development of cor pulmonale are also predictive of outcome[137,150,151] (*see Fig. 3.4 and Box 3.7*).

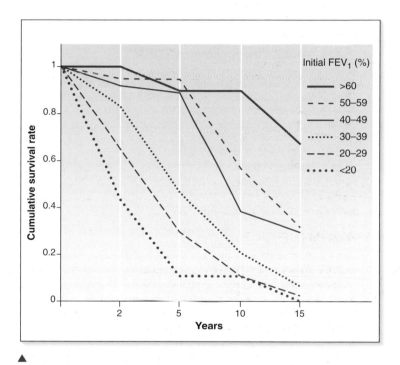

Fig. 3.4 The relationship between FEV_1 and survival in COPD. (From Traver et al.[137])

BOX 3.7 Factors that predict outcome in COPD

■ FEV_1
■ Breathlessness on MRC scale
■ Exercise capacity
■ Body mass index
■ Total lung diffusion capacity (T_LCO)
■ PaO_2
■ Cor pulmonale
■ Health status

PATIENT QUESTIONS

3.35   Will I get better?

Unfortunately the damage caused to the lungs in COPD does not go away. Stopping smoking prevents the accelerated decline in lung function seen in smokers but so far no treatment has been shown to affect the progression of the disease.

3.36   What are the symptoms of COPD?

The commonest symptoms are breathlessness on exertion (e.g. climbing hills or stairs), a cough (which may be productive of white or green sputum) and exacerbations (which may appear to be chest infections or episodes of bronchitis and which often occur in the winter). Other symptoms are wheezing, chest pain, ankle swelling, weight loss and feeling depressed.

3.37   How is COPD diagnosed?

COPD is often diagnosed solely on the basis of a patient's symptoms and the fact that they have smoked. To make an accurate diagnosis of COPD it is necessary to show that there is narrowing of the airways and that the narrowing does not change much either from day to day or in response to treatment. This is best done by performing a breathing test called spirometry. Sometimes this is done before and after a trial of treatment with bronchodilator or steroid medication.

3.38   What is spirometry?

Spirometry is a way of measuring the amount of air exhaled from the lungs. It is usual to measure the total amount of air exhaled after taking in as deep a breath as possible (this is known as the vital capacity). The exhalation is usually done using maximum effort, in which case the amount of air exhaled is known as the forced vital capacity (FVC) but it can also be done gently in which case the amount exhaled is known as the slow vital capacity (slow VC). Spirometry also measures the amount of air exhaled in the first second (this is known as the forced expiratory volume in 1 second or FEV_1). If there is narrowing of the airways less air is exhaled in the first second and so the FEV_1 and the FEV_1 as a proportion of the FVC are reduced.

Management guidelines for COPD

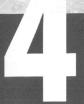

4.1 What guidelines exist to assist the treatment of COPD?

Guidelines on the management of COPD were published by the British Thoracic Society (BTS) in 1997.[152] North American guidelines on the management of COPD[153] and a European Consensus Statement[154] were published in 1995. These are all under revision, but the latest COPD guidelines come from the Global Initiative for Chronic Obstructive Lung Disease (GOLD).[155] This initiative was established by the US National Heart, Lung and Blood Institute (NHLBI) in conjunction with the World Health Organization (WHO). Its goals are 'to increase awareness of COPD and decrease mortality and morbidity' from COPD by encouraging research and making consensus-based recommendations on management of COPD.

4.2 How can the effects of treatments be assessed?

Traditionally, the effects of interventions have been assessed by measuring changes in the FEV_1 but, by definition, there is limited scope for this to change and other outcome measures must be considered (*Box 4.1*). Other spirometric indices such as the slow vital capacity (SVC) and inspiratory capacity (IC) may correlate better with the clinical response to therapy.[156] Improvements in patient-centred outcomes such as symptoms, exercise capacity and health status may occur without significant changes in FEV_1,[157] and reductions in the frequency of exacerbations may also be relevant.

4.3 How can the effects of treatments be assessed in routine clinical practice?

Many of the measures used in clinical trials are too cumbersome or time consuming to be used on a routine basis in primary care. As discussed above, relying on changes in spirometry may miss clinically significant changes. Adequate information about improvements may be obtained by asking simple questions such as:

BOX 4.1 Outcome measures in COPD

- Spirometry
- Walking distance
- Dyspnoea indices
- Symptom scores
- Health status
- Exacerbation rate

■ Has your treatment made a difference to you?
■ Is your breathing easier in any way?
■ Can you do some things now that you could not do at all before the treatment, or do you do the same things but faster?
■ Can you do the same things as before but are now less breathless when you do them?

4.4   What are the aims of treatment of patients with stable COPD?

Attempts should be made to diagnose patients as early in the course of their disease as possible and it is important that the diagnosis should be accurate. When managing patients with stable COPD treatment should aim to give the best control of symptoms, to improve patients' ability to undertake activities of daily living, to improve health-related quality of life, to prevent disease progression and complications and to reduce mortality. It is also important to ensure that the patient has optimal support and education to help them cope with their disease.

 PATIENT QUESTIONS

4.5   Has anyone laid down national standards for the treatment of COPD?

Guidelines for doctors and nurses on the management of COPD were produced by the British Thoracic Society in 1997. These still contain many important messages, but they do not discuss some of the treatments that have become available in the last few years. Within the UK the Department of Health has asked the National Institute for Clinical Excellence (NICE) to produce new guidelines and it is expected that these will be published early in 2004.

Prevention of COPD

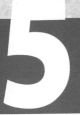

5.1 Can COPD be prevented?

Stopping patients smoking is the single most effective way of altering the outcome in patients at all stages in COPD. This is as true for presymptomatic patients with airflow obstruction as it is for patients with severe disease. Those who continue to smoke will continue to lose FEV_1 at an accelerated rate, and although lost function cannot be regained, those who stop smoking will deteriorate more slowly and derive more benefit from therapies such as oxygen.

Stopping smoking returns the accelerated rate of decline in FEV_1 seen in smokers back to the normal rate[158] and smokers with airflow limitation benefit from quitting despite previous heavy smoking, advanced age or poor baseline lung function[159] (*Fig. 5.1*). Workers in dusty occupations associated with the development of COPD should be strongly advised not to smoke and they should be provided with, and wear, appropriate and effective respiratory protection in the workplace.

5.2 What methods of smoking cessation can be used?

Smoking cessation is an extremely cost-effective intervention.[160,161] It can be very satisfying for those involved and offers significant cardiovascular benefits as well as offering the potential to prevent the development of COPD.

Advice about stopping smoking should be given at every opportunity. Successful quitters consistently list advice from a health professional as one of the main motivational factors for stopping smokers and even brief advice can significantly improve quit rates.

Basic anti-smoking advice should be given to all smokers as part of an integrated service offering counselling and support.[162] Recent advances in the pharmacotherapy of nicotine addiction have led to significantly higher quit rates[163] and bupropion has been shown to be effective in patients with COPD.[164]

5.3 Does making a diagnosis of COPD affect the success of smoking cessation?

A number of studies have shown that demonstrating to patients that their lungs have already been damaged by smoking by performing spirometry improves quit rates. This was shown in a number of early studies,[165,166] but recently a Norwegian study showed that informing men aged 30–45 if they had a low FEV_1 improved self-reported sustained 12 month quit rates from 3.5 to 5.6%.[167] A large Polish study has also shown similar benefits.[168]

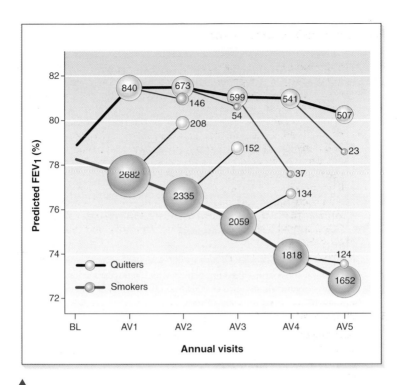

▲
Fig. 5.1 Lung function changes in quitters and continuing smokers. (From Scanlon et al.[159])

5.4   Do drugs help patients with COPD to stop smoking?

Pharmacotherapy using nicotine replacement improves quit rates and bupropion, particularly when used in conjunction with psychological support, can result in sustained cessation for 12 months in around 25% of smokers. In patients with COPD sustained cessation rates at 6 months are around 16%.[164]

5.5   Can alpha-1 antitrypsin (α-1 AT) deficiency be prevented?

There are conflicting views about whether the relatives of a patient with α-1 AT deficiency should be screened for α-1 AT deficiency themselves[169] (*see also Ch. 14*). The main point of identifying asymptomatic family members is to ensure that they do not smoke as replacement therapy is of unproven benefit.

PATIENT QUESTIONS

5.6 Can anything be done to prevent COPD?

COPD is very uncommon in non-smokers and in people who are not exposed to passive cigarette smoke. Avoiding smoking and wearing adequate respiratory protection (i.e. masks) if working in dusty occupations are the best ways of preventing COPD.

5.7 Will I get better if I stop smoking?

Stopping smoking will prevent further damage to the lungs. Unfortunately, stopping smoking cannot undo the damage that has already been done, but stopping smoking may allow certain treatments, particularly oxygen, to work more effectively.

5.8 How can I stop smoking?

There are now many ways your doctor can help you to stop smoking. These range from advice and support to the prescription of nicotine replacement therapy and a drug called bupropion which reduces the desire to smoke. Many organizations, such as ASH and QUIT (*see Ch. 14*) also provide help and advice about stopping smoking.

Drug therapy

6.1 What is the role of bronchodilators in COPD?

Although the disease is characterized by substantially irreversible airflow obstruction, bronchodilators are still the mainstay of pharmacotherapy.[170,171] Beta agonists, anticholinergics and theophylline are all effective bronchodilators in COPD. The choice of therapy depends on individual responses.

SHORT-ACTING BETA AGONISTS

6.2 How do short-acting beta agonists work?

Beta agonists act directly on bronchial smooth muscle to cause bronchodilatation. They are the most widely used bronchodilators for COPD. The dose response relationship for salbutamol in patients with largely or completely irreversible COPD is almost flat.[172,173] The time to peak response is slower than in asthmatics and the side-effect to benefits ratio is such that there is little benefit in giving more than 1 mg salbutamol. They are effective for up to 4 hours and can be used both on a regular, or as required, basis (*Box 6.1*).

6.3 What are the indications for their use?

Short-acting beta agonists are widely used as first line therapy for patients with COPD either on an as-needed or regular basis. They are often used in combination with anticholinergic bronchodilators.

6.4 What is the evidence base for their use?

Although many of the early studies included relatively few subjects and were of short duration, there is a good body of evidence to support the use of short-acting beta agonists. Much of this has been the subject of a review by the Cochrane Airways Group.[174] Studies comparing short-acting beta agonist with placebo have shown significant increases in FEV_1, peak expiratory flow (PEF) rates and symptom scores.[174] Patients who do not

---

BOX 6.1 Effects of short-acting beta agonists

■ Increased FEV_1
■ Reduced breathlessness
■ Increased exercise capacity
■ Improved health status

have a significant spirometric response may still benefit if alternative outcome measures such as walking distances are assessed. Beta agonists do not have any significant effect on cough or sputum production, and their effects on walking distance have been inconsistent.

6.5   What are their adverse effects?

 Short-acting beta agonists may produce adverse effects that are related to the pharmacological actions of the drugs as well as effects that are due to long term administration and idiosyncratic effects.[175]

■ Adverse effects due to the pharmacological properties are uncommon when beta agonists are administered by the inhaled route. The main effect is tremor due to effects on skeletal muscle[176] but occasionally tachycardia may occur.[177] Beta agonists may also produce transient hypoxia by worsening ventilation perfusion matching[178] and this may be relevant in patients treated with high doses at the time of an exacerbation. They also produce acute hyperglycaemia, hypokalaemia and hypomagnesaemia.[175] Hypokalaemia may contribute to the development of dysrhythmias in hypoxic patients at the time of exacerbations (*see also Q. 7.13*).

■ Long term administration of beta agonists in asthmatics may lead to the development of tolerance[176] and this may lead to a shortening of the duration of bronchodilatation.[179,180] It is likely that similar effects will occur in patients with COPD. There have been occasional reports of severe bronchospasm immediately after the inhalation of short-acting beta agonists.[181] Some of these may be due to other components of the aerosol.

SHORT-ACTING ANTICHOLINERGICS

6.6   How do short-acting anticholinergics work?

Cholinergic nerves are the main neural bronchoconstrictor pathway in the airways and the resting tone is increased in patients with COPD.[182] Anticholinergic drugs cause bronchodilatation by blocking this bronchoconstrictor effect.

Cholinergic effects on the airway are mediated by muscarinic receptors and these also mediate effects on mucus secretion. Three muscarinic receptors are now recognized: M1 mediate cholinergic transmission in parasympathetic ganglia, M2 mediate feedback inhibition of acetylcholine (ACh) release from preganglionic nerves and M3 mediate smooth muscle contraction. Effective anticholinergic drugs block M1 and M3 receptors in preference to M2 receptors.[183]

6.7 What are the indications for their use?

As increased cholinergic tone is the principal reversible mechanism of airway obstruction in COPD, short-acting anticholinergics should be the first choice bronchodilator in patients with COPD; however, they are often used after patients have been prescribed short-acting beta agonists. The optimal dose of ipratropium is around 80 μg, which is higher than the dose usually prescribed.[184]

6.8 What is the evidence base for their use?

There is a good body of evidence to support the use of short-acting anticholinergic bronchodilators. Ipratropium and oxitropium produce more sustained bronchodilatation (up to 8 hours) than short-acting beta agonists and are possibly more effective,[185–187] but the speed of onset of action of is slower. Unlike the beta agonists, anticholinergic bronchodilators have also been shown to have a beneficial effect on sleep quality in patients with COPD.[188]

6.9 What are their adverse effects?

 Short-acting anticholinergics may produce adverse effects that are related to the pharmacological actions of the drugs as well as idiosyncratic effects.[189] There is no evidence of the development of effects due to long term administration.

- Adverse effects due to the pharmacological properties of short-acting anticholinergics are uncommon when they are administered by the inhaled route. The main effect is dry mouth due to inhibition of muscarinic stimulation of salivary secretion. Ipratropium does not appear to have any significant effect on airway mucus or mucociliary clearance.[189]
- Ocular effects – particularly raised intraocular pressure, difficulty with accommodation and narrow angle glaucoma – have been reported in patients using nebulised short-acting anticholinergics due to a direct contact of the aerosol with the cornea but this is not seen with the metered dose inhaler preparation unless it is sprayed directly into the eye.[189]
- Unlike the short-acting beta agonists, ipratropium has no effect on ventilation perfusion matching.[190]
- There have been occasional reports of severe bronchospasm immediately after the inhalation of short-acting anticholinergics.[191] Some of these may be due to other components of the aerosol.

LONG-ACTING BETA AGONISTS

6.10 How do long-acting beta agonists work?

The bronchodilator effects of long-acting beta agonists are similar to the short-acting agents but their duration of action is around 12 hours. They may have additional effects on intracellular cyclic adenosine monophosphate (cAMP) levels and in in-vitro models, and in normal subjects may have effects on mucociliary clearance and bacterial adherence.[192] The importance of these effects in COPD is not known.

6.11 What are the indications for their use?

Long-acting beta agonists are effective drugs which are indicated in patients who remain symptomatic despite using short-acting bronchodilators. Extrapolating from the evidence regarding short-acting drugs, it seems likely that they may offer benefits if combined with an anticholinergic. Long-acting beta agonists are more expensive than short-acting drugs but in patients who respond they are more convenient.

6.12 What is the evidence base for their use?

Some patients with COPD undoubtedly get symptomatic benefit. Studies have shown that they produce improvements of approximately 100–200 ml in FEV_1 and they improve health status and breathlessness scores.[193–197] These effects are dose dependent and maximum improvement in health status is produced by salmeterol 50 µg or formoterol (eformoterol) 12 µg twice daily.[196,197] Larger doses have a reduced effect.

Long-acting beta agonists appear to reduce exacerbation rates in COPD (*see Q. 7.5*) but the mechanism responsible for this remains unclear. Effects on host defences have been proposed[192] but it is possible that the effects are due to a reduction in baseline breathlessness which leads to reduced recognition of exacerbations as a result of increased tolerance of the increased breathlessness that occurs (*see Box 6.2*).

BOX 6.2 Effects of long-acting beta agonists

■ Improved FEV_1
■ Reduced symptoms
■ Increased exercise tolerance
■ Improved health status
■ Reduced exacerbation rate

6.13 Are there differences between drugs in this class?

Salmeterol has a slower onset of action than formoterol (eformoterol).
There are no other clinically relevant differences between the molecules.
Studies on the effects of formoterol (eformoterol) in COPD have shown
more consistent results than those on salmeterol.

6.14 What are their adverse effects?

 Like the short-acting beta agonists, long-acting beta agonists may
produce adverse effects that are related to the pharmacological actions
of the drugs: tremor, tachycardia and hypokalaemia. Because of the
increased duration of action, these effects limit the use of such drugs in
some patients.

There has been concern that these drugs may induce cardiac
dysrhythmias in patients with COPD but there is no evidence that this is a
problem in practice.[198]

Transient paradoxical bronchospasm has been reported in asthmatic
patients treated with salmeterol.[199] There is also evidence that the maximum
bronchodilator response to salmeterol is reduced after 6 months of use.[200]
This may be due to β_2 receptor downregulation.

LONG-ACTING ANTICHOLINERGICS

6.15 How do long-acting anticholinergics work?

There is currently only one long-acting anticholinergic bronchodilator
available. This is given once daily[201] and has kinetic selectivity for M1
and M3 receptors.[202] Studies have suggested that it has effects that are
both qualitatively and quantitatively different to the regular use of
short-acting anticholinergics. The mechanisms underlying this are still
not clear.

6.16 What are the indications for their use?

> Tiotropium is an effective drug which is indicated in patients who
> remain symptomatic despite using short-acting bronchodilators.
> Extrapolating from the evidence regarding short-acting drugs, it
> seems likely that there may be additional benefits if it is combined
> with a beta agonist; however, the magnitude of such additional
> benefits would have to be balanced against the additional cost of
> combination therapy.

6.17 What is the evidence base for their use?

The use of tiotropium is supported by randomized controlled trial over 12 months comparing its effects with those of placebo or ipratropium. It has also been shown to be more effective than salmeterol in a study lasting 6 months. These studies have shown that it is an effective bronchodilator in that it reduces breathlessness, improves exercise tolerance, reduces exacerbations and improves health status.[201,203,204]

6.18 What are their adverse effects?

Dry mouth is the main adverse effect of long-acting anticholinergic therapy. Like the short-acting drugs, this is due to inhibition of muscarinic stimulation of salivary secretion. To date no other significant adverse events have been reported.

INHALED STEROIDS

6.19 How do inhaled steroids work?

There is little evidence that inhaled steroids have any effects on the inflammatory cells present in COPD: neutrophils, unlike eosinophils, are relatively insensitive to the effects of steroids. Even high doses of inhaled steroids do not reduce the number of inflammatory cells or the levels of cytokines.[205,206] However, there are clinical data which show a reduction in exacerbation rates (see Q. 7.5) in patients treated with inhaled steroids. The mechanisms by which these effects are achieved are still unclear.

6.20 What are the indications for their use?

The role of inhaled steroids in stable COPD is controversial. On the basis of current evidence it appears that the principal indication for inhaled steroids is in patients with severe COPD (FEV_1 < 40% predicted) who are having frequent exacerbations (see Qs 7.13 and 7.16). They may also have a role in potentiating the effects of long-acting beta agonists. They do not affect the rate of decline in lung function.

6.21 What is the evidence base for their use?

The role of inhaled steroids in stable COPD (*Box 6.3*) has been the subject of four recent large trials.[207–210] All used changes in the rate of decline in FEV_1 as the primary endpoint and showed no benefit. Inhaled steroids appear to reduce the number of exacerbations in patients with severe

---

> **BOX 6.3 Role of inhaled steroids**
> ■ No effect on disease progression
> ■ May reduce exacerbation rates in patients with severe disease
> ■ May slow rate of decline in health status

COPD[207,208,211] and this may be the main benefit of treatment (*see also Qs 7.13 and 7.16*).

6.22 What are their adverse effects?

 High dose inhaled steroids in patients with COPD may reduce bone mineral density.[208] They may also be associated with oral candidiasis and dysphonia, and skin thinning and easy bruising in susceptible patients. The benefits must be balanced against such side-effects.[212]

6.23 Are there differences between drugs in this class?

There is no evidence and no pharmacological reason to suggest that different steroid molecules have different effects in COPD.

ORAL STEROIDS

6.24 What are the indications for their use?

Trials of oral steroid therapy can help to identify patients with a significant untreated chronic asthmatic component to their disease[213] who may benefit from being managed according to asthma protocols, but they are poor predictors of response to inhaled steroids in patients with COPD.[214] The vast majority of patients with COPD can be managed without regular oral steroid therapy; however, a small proportion of patients do appear to deteriorate if low dose (usually less than 5 mg per day) maintenance therapy with oral steroids is withdrawn. These patients must be warned about the risks of developing osteoporosis and should be offered effective therapy to reduce this risk.

The role of oral steroids (*Box 6.4*) in the management of acute exacerbations is discussed later (*see Q.7.17*).

6.25 What is the evidence base for their use?

At best, trials of oral corticosteroids in patients with stable disease have shown improvements in small subsets (15–40%);[215] however, this may be achieved at considerable cost in terms of side-effects and at present there is

> **BOX 6.4 Role of oral steroids**
>
> ■ Identify patients with significant asthmatic component
> ■ Speed recovery from an exacerbation
> ■ Delay time to next exacerbation
> ■ Produce sustained reduction in symptoms in a very small proportion
>   of patients

no means of predicting those who will respond positively. Less than half of those patients who show objective improvements with oral therapy maintain the improvement on inhaled corticosteroid therapy.[216]

6.26 What are their adverse effects?

Oral steroids carry with them a dose- and duration-dependent risk of systemic side-effects.[212] There is some individual variability in the susceptibility to the development of side-effects. Patients may notice increased appetite, fluid retention and mood swings with short term treatment. With longer term, high dose treatment patients may develop skin thinning, easy bruising, weight gain, osteoporosis, cataracts, proximal myopathy, diabetes and hypertension. Patients should be made aware of these effects and when appropriate they should be prescribed therapy (such as hormone or bisphosphonate therapy) to reduce the risk of osteoporosis.

COMBINATION THERAPY: BETA AGONISTS AND ANTICHOLINERGICS

6.27 How do combinations of beta agonists and anticholinergics work?

By both blocking the increased resting cholinergic tone and directly relaxing airway smooth muscle, giving short-acting beta agonists at the same time as anticholinergic bronchodilators leads to greater increases in FEV_1, or other measures of airway calibre, than either drug alone.[217–220] Used in this way greater bronchodilatation can be achieved with fewer side-effects.

6.28 What are the indications for their use?

Until recently, combinations of short-acting beta agonists and anticholinergics were the mainstay of bronchodilator therapy in COPD. They remain a useful and cost effective first line treatment for some patients but the introduction of the long-acting bronchodilators, particularly tiotropium, has limited their indications in patients who remain symptomatic. Combination therapy may produce greater symptom relief with fewer side-effects than increasing the dose of a single agent, but may be more expensive. Inhalers containing combinations of ipratropium and salbutamol are also available and offer greater convenience.[187] It is worth trying combinations of short-acting beta agonists and anticholinergics in patients with mild symptoms, but if these are not adequately controlled and if patients continue to experience limitations on their activities of daily living, a long-acting bronchodilator should be tried.

6.29 What is the evidence base for their use?

The use of combinations of short-acting beta agonists and anticholinergics has been shown to be effective in in-vitro models, in short-term physiological studies[187,219,221,222] and in clinical trials.

6.30 What are their adverse effects?

 Information on adverse effects can be found under the individual drugs outlined above. There are no additional adverse effects from using such drugs in combination.

COMBINATION THERAPY: BRONCHODILATORS AND STEROIDS

6.31 How do combinations of long-acting beta agonists and steroids work?

A number of mechanisms have been proposed to explain the apparent synergy between inhaled long-acting beta agonists and steroids. None of these has been shown convincingly to be the mechanism responsible for the effect. An effect of the steroids on beta receptor numbers or post-receptor mechanism is the most plausible explanation, but there are data which suggest that salmeterol may have synergistic effects with steroids on inflammatory cells.

6.32 What are the indications for their use?

Combinations of inhaled long-acting beta agonists and steroids may provide an alternative to the use of a long-acting anticholinergic in patients who remain symptomatic despite using a combination of short-acting bronchodilators.

6.33 What is the evidence base for their use?

A number of studies looking at the clinical effects of combinations of long-acting beta agonists and corticosteroids have been presented in abstract form[223–228] and are beginning to be published.[229,230] There are a number of studies using in-vitro models or normal volunteers looking at possible explanations for the apparent interactions.[192]

6.34 What are their adverse effects?

Information on adverse effects can be found under the individual drugs outlined above. There are no additional adverse effects from using such drugs in combination.

THEOPHYLLINES

6.35 How do theophyllines work?

Theophylline belongs to a class of drugs known as methylxanthines. The mechanism of action of methylxanthines remains uncertain.[231,232] Their primary effect is generally assumed to be relaxation of airway smooth muscle; however, at therapeutic concentrations they have limited bronchodilator effect.[233] Theophylline also appears to increase diaphragmatic strength in patients with COPD[234] and this may improve ventilation and delay the onset of fatigue. Theophylline has effects on mucociliary clearance,[235] as well as extrapulmonary effects (particularly improvement in cardiac output[236]) that may also be beneficial in patients with COPD.

Theophyllines also appear to increase respiratory drive[237,238] and this appears capable of overcoming some of the respiratory depression present during exacerbations.[239]

6.36 What are the indications for their use?

Sustained release oral theophylline and aminophylline produce symptomatic relief and improvements in FEV_1.[240–242] They appear to be less effective than long-acting beta agonists[243] and as such are now usually reserved as third line therapy, usually in combination with inhaled therapy.[244] Because of potential toxicity and significant interactions with other drugs,[245] they require monitoring of plasma concentrations[246] (*Box 6.5*).

Theophyllines are used in COPD but their use is declining.[247]

BOX 6.5 Theophylline

■ Used third line when patients fail to respond to inhaled beta agonists and anticholinergics

■ Side-effects (nausea and tachycardia) may be problematic

■ Plasma concentrations need monitoring

■ Plasma levels are affected by concomitant therapy and smoking

6.37 What is the evidence base for their use?

A systematic review of oral theophylline identified 20 appropriately designed and reported studies that examined the effects of oral theophylline in COPD.[248] All were of a crossover design with adequate washout periods, but their duration was short, the longest being 90 days. Thirteen studies reported changes in FEV$_1$ and showed significant improvements, 11 also reported changes in forced vital capacity (FVC) and again showed significant improvements. The two studies that looked at 6 minute walking distance showed no significant changes.[240,249] Those studies that reported nausea rates showed that they were significantly higher in patients taking theophylline (relative risk 7.67).[248]

6.38 What are their adverse effects?

The therapeutic index of theophylline is narrow and some patients experience significant side-effects even when the plasma levels are in the therapeutic range. Rapid increases in plasma levels even within the therapeutic range are more likely to produce adverse events.[246] Approximately 5% of patients develop unacceptable side-effects when the plasma concentrations are above 80 μmol/l and serious adverse reactions (persistent vomiting, gastrointestinal bleeding, fits, cardiac arrhythmias and cardiorespiratory arrest) often occur at concentrations above 110 μmol/l. Ageing associated changes in liver function lead to a greater risk of toxicity in the elderly.[250]

6.39 How often should plasma levels be monitored?

For most patients a measurement of plasma theophylline concentrations 8–10 hours following a single oral dose will be sufficient to predict maintenance requirements and a repeat measurement 1–2 weeks later will confirm that the plasma concentration is in the therapeutic range. Thereafter, monitoring is not necessary unless there has been a change in either concomitant medication or the patient's condition that would lead to altered theophylline clearance.[246]

6.40 What is the difference between theophylline and aminophylline?

Theophylline is the pharmacologically active molecule but since it is only slightly soluble in water, it is difficult to administer. Aminophylline is a combination of theophylline and ethylenediamine and is the most commonly used of the theophylline salts. It increases the amount of available theophylline around 20-fold.

INHALATION SYSTEMS

6.41 Does the type of inhaler matter?

As with asthma, delivery of the drugs to the lungs is an essential part of pharmacotherapy. When considering delivery devices, coexisting problems (e.g. arthritis) must be taken into account (*Box 6.6*). Pressurized metered dose inhalers (pMDIs) are cheap but unless used with large volume spacers give poor pulmonary deposition and up to 75% of patients with COPD are unable to use them correctly.[251] Dry powder devices are more expensive but can be used successfully by around 90% of patients and thus may be significantly more cost effective. Many elderly patients soon forget how to use their inhalers correctly[252] and it is essential to check their inhaler technique at every opportunity and re-instruct as necessary.

6.42 When should large volume spacers be used?

The use of large volume spacers with metered dose inhalers is a well-established method of maximizing pulmonary drug deposition in patients with asthma, but there have been few studies in COPD. Poor coordination may significantly impair an elderly patient's ability to use a metered dose inhaler and this can be improved using a large volume spacer.[251]

6.43 What is a nebuliser?

Nebulisers are devices that generate a mist of aqueous particles that are small enough to be inhaled and reach the airways. They are usually driven by compressed air generated by an electrical pump but they can also be driven by compressed air or oxygen from cylinders (*Fig. 6.1*). Most patients achieve maximum possible bronchodilatation with drugs administered by conventional inhalers, but a few derive benefit from very high doses of bronchodilating drugs.[253,254] These high doses are most conveniently delivered using a nebuliser. Compressors to drive nebulisers are relatively cheap, but the drug costs are high and patients may experience more severe systemic effects.

BOX 6.6 Factors affecting choice of delivery systems

■ Dexterity
■ Hand grip strength
■ Coordination
■ Severity of airflow limitation

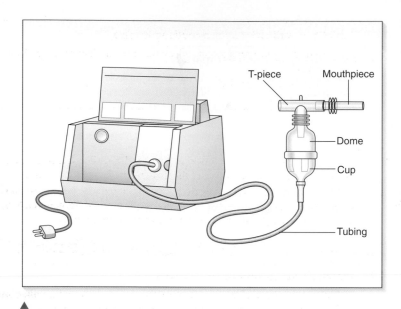

▲

Fig. 6.1 A nebuliser and compressor.

6.44 What are the indications for nebulised therapy?

There is conflicting evidence about whether there is any advantage in delivering the same doses of drugs by inhaler or nebuliser.[255–259] A few patients do appear to derive additional benefits from nebulised therapy, but before recommending that they use nebulisers on a regular basis, these patients should have tried maximal doses of inhaled therapy, have had a trial of oral steroids and have a formal assessment of the efficacy of nebulised therapy.[260] It is important to realize that there may be a strong placebo effect and that some patients appear to benefit from the moistening or cooling effects of the aerosol generated by a nebuliser, rather than by the drugs they deliver. Nebulised therapy may also be indicated at the time of exacerbations (see Q. 7.14). Indications for nebulised therapy are outlined in Box 6.7.

6.45 How can the effects of nebulised therapy be assessed?

In the UK, the British Thoracic Society (BTS) nebuliser guidelines make recommendations about the assessment of patients for nebuliser therapy[260] (see also Ch. 14). As discussed earlier, patients may derive significant symptomatic benefit from nebulised therapy compared with inhaled

BOX 6.7 Indications for nebulised therapy

■ Persistent symptoms despite adequate bronchodilator therapy from inhalers
■ Inability to use inhalers
■ Exacerbations

therapy without having a significant change in FEV_1. This limits the value of objective assessments of nebuliser therapy and the best assessment may simply be to ask the patients whether they are able to do more or whether they have fewer symptoms as a result of using nebulised bronchodilators, and whether or not they have experienced any adverse effects.

MANAGEMENT

6.46 Which drugs should be used first line?

Although long-acting drugs give better symptom control, reduce disability by improving exercise capacity and reduce exacerbation rates (see Q. 7.5), it is still appropriate to start patients with mild disease on regular plus 'as needed' short-acting drugs either alone or in combination. Patients who remain symptomatic or those with more severe disease will get better control, experience fewer symptoms, and have less disability if they are prescribed a long-acting bronchodilator.

6.47 Which drug combinations are effective?

Combinations of short-acting anticholinergics and beta agonists have been shown to be more effective than either component alone.[217-220] Whether the same holds true for the long-acting drugs is not yet known. Combinations of inhaled steroids and long-acting beta agonists seem more effective than the long-acting beta agonists alone[229,230] and adding theophylline to a long-acting beta agonist also seems more effective than either component alone.[261]

6.48 Are fixed combinations useful?

A fixed combination of a short-acting anticholinergic and a beta agonist in the same inhaler has been available for some years; this offers convenience for the patient and reduces prescription costs.[187] However, it does limit the use of the short-acting beta agonist as rescue medication and patients may need an additional inhaler for this. Fixed combinations of inhaled steroids and long-acting beta agonists may also offer advantages in terms of cost and convenience and in this case it is unlikely that patients would need to use variable doses of one of the components.

BOX 6.8 Indications for referral

■ Diagnostic uncertainty
■ Disproportionate symptoms
■ Persistent symptoms
■ Development of lung cancer
■ Pulmonary rehabilitation
■ Nebuliser assessment
■ Oxygen assessment
■ Surgical opinion

6.49 Which patients should be referred to hospital?

Most patients with COPD can be managed in primary care but some may require referral to a specialist. This may be because of diagnostic uncertainty, the presence of symptoms that seem out of proportion to the measured lung function abnormality, or for advice on management of persistent symptoms. Patients who have symptoms suggestive of the development of lung cancer (e.g. haemoptysis or weight loss) should be referred urgently. Patients may need to be referred for pulmonary rehabilitation, for assessment of their requirement for nebulised bronchodilator therapy or the need for oxygen therapy. Indications for hospital referral are summarized in *Box 6.8.*

 PATIENT QUESTIONS

6.50 How is COPD treated?

The treatment for COPD depends on which symptoms are present and the extent of lung damage. Many patients only need treatment at the time of an exacerbation and this is often simply a course of antibiotics (*see Qs 7.13, 7.16 and 7.19*) . Patients with regular symptoms usually need to inhale drugs that relax the muscle in the walls of the airways and reduce the narrowing that is present. Patients who have severe narrowing of the airways and who are having frequent exacerbations may also be prescribed a steroid inhaler to try to reduce the frequency of exacerbations (*see Q. 7.13*). In more advanced cases patients may be given extra oxygen to breathe, either in short bursts to relieve symptoms or continuously for at least 16 hours per day. Some patients need courses of steroid tablets at the time of an exacerbation and a few patients are prescribed regular steroid tablets (*see Qs 7.13 and 7.16*).

6.51   Do I have to have steroids?

Inhaled steroids have been shown to reduce the frequency of exacerbations in patients with advanced COPD (*see Qs 7.13 and 7.16*). Their role in milder disease is less clear. Steroid tablets have been shown to speed the recovery of patients admitted to hospital with an exacerbation and delay the development of future exacerbations. They appear to have similar benefits when used to treat exacerbations in patients not admitted to hospital. Their benefits when used as regular, daily treatment are less clear but some patients do seem to derive benefit and appear to deteriorate if the dose is reduced or if the tablets are stopped.

6.52   Do I need a nebuliser?

Nebulisers are simply devices that deliver high doses of drugs to the lung in a mist form. They are operated by air from a compressor. Most patients can be treated using inhalers; however, a few patients benefit from the higher doses of drugs used in nebulisers and some may also benefit from the cooling effect of the particles and the fact that less effort is needed to inhale the drugs than if inhalers are used.

6.53   Will I need to go to hospital?

Many patients with COPD are treated in the community but some will be referred to hospital. There are a number of reasons why patients are referred, including the need for a specialist opinion, to have their requirements for oxygen or nebulised therapy assessed, or for treatment of exacerbations.

Treating exacerbations of COPD

7

PQ PATIENT QUESTIONS

7.1　What is an exacerbation of COPD?

Exacerbations are one of the most important features of COPD. They occur in patients at all stages of their disease but are most common in those with severe disease. Many mild exacerbations are not reported by patients to their general practitioner/primary care physician (GP/PCP),[262] but for many patients exacerbations are the only occasions when they consider themselves to have an illness and the only occasions on which they consult their GP/PCP. Exacerbations manifest as a worsening of existing symptoms and patients frequently believe that they have an 'infection'.

7.2　What causes exacerbations?

Many exacerbations are related to infections, both viral and bacterial, but inhalation of air pollutants and changes in the weather may also be important.[263,264] The most common pathogens identified in patients at the time of exacerbations are *Haemophilus influenzae, Streptococcus pneumoniae* and *Moraxella catarrhalis,* but these organisms can also be isolated from the sputum of patients with stable disease and their role in causing exacerbations is still unclear.[265,266] Other pathogens such as *Chlamydia pneumoniae* may also be important.

7.3　Are some patients at greater risk of exacerbations?

Evidence suggests that exacerbations become more frequent as patients' lung function declines. Patients who experience three or more exacerbations per year are also at risk of continuing to have frequent exacerbations.

An increased risk of hospital admission with an exacerbation has also been shown to be associated with the underprescription of home oxygen in patients who meet the criteria for long term oxygen therapy, the underuse of influenza vaccination, the underuse of pulmonary rehabilitation, poor inhaler technique and continued active or passive smoking.[267]

7.4　What are the consequences of having an exacerbation?

Exacerbations are an important determinant of adverse health status. Most patients make a full recovery from an exacerbation within 1 week, but some patients experiencing frequent exacerbations take longer to recover. A few patients have not made a full recovery and their lung function has not returned to the pre-exacerbation level by the time the next exacerbation occurs. For these patients exacerbations are an important cause of progressive deterioration. Exacerbations may also be the final factor that leads to patients losing the ability to live independently.

7.5 Can exacerbations be prevented?

A number of recent studies have shown that inhaled steroids and long-acting bronchodilators reduce exacerbation rates.[268-271] These effects may be due to reducing airway inflammation (in the case of steroids) or by improving background levels of breathlessness, thereby reducing patients' perception of the increased symptoms at the time of exacerbations.

Vaccination may help to prevent exacerbations by reducing the risk of influenza infections.

7.6 What are the symptoms of an exacerbation?

Increased breathlessness is the commonest symptom of an exacerbation. Change in sputum colour (with increased purulence and increased sputum volume) and wheeze are also common symptoms. Some patients also experience sore throats or symptoms of colds and some will develop worsening ankle swelling. Symptoms of an exacerbation are summarized in *Box. 7.1.*

7.7 How can exacerbations be diagnosed?

Exacerbations can usually be diagnosed on the basis of the symptoms. Many mild exacerbations are self-diagnosed and managed: patients simply use more of their maintenance bronchodilators to control symptoms.[262]

7.8 What other conditions may present with similar features to an exacerbation of COPD?

The differential diagnosis of a worsening of symptoms includes cardiac dysfunction, pneumonia, pulmonary emboli, a pneumothorax and bronchial obstruction due to a tumour (*Box 7.2*). Without a chest radiograph it is difficult to differentiate an exacerbation of COPD from pneumonia but in practice most of these patients will meet the criteria suggested for referral to hospital and a radiograph will be obtained.

BOX 7.1 Symptoms of an exacerbation

■ Increased breathlessness
■ Increased sputum volume
■ Increased sputum purulence
■ Wheeze
■ Ankle swelling
■ Symptoms of a cold
■ Fever or rigors

BOX 7.2 Differential diagnosis of an exacerbation

- Pulmonary embolus
- Pneumothorax
- Myocardial infarction
- Left ventricular failure
- Pneumonia
- Bronchial carcinoma

7.9 What investigations are needed during exacerbations?

Investigations are not usually required when managing exacerbations at home. Sputum culture is of little value and blood tests are not usually indicated. If it is available, pulse oximetry can identify patients who are hypoxic and who need referral to hospital.

7.10 Which patients with exacerbations need referring to hospital?

Most patients can be managed at home but a few need hospital treatment. COPD guidelines (e.g. those of the British Thoracic Society, BTS; *see Ch. 14*) make recommendations about factors to consider when deciding where to treat patients (*Box 7.3*). Essentially the decision involves an assessment of the severity of symptoms (particularly the degree of breathlessness, the presence of cyanosis or peripheral oedema and the level of consciousness), the presence of comorbidities, whether or not the patient is already receiving long term oxygen therapy, the level of physical functioning, and the patient's ability to cope at home.

BOX 7.3 Factors favouring referral to hospital for management of an exacerbation

- Unable to cope at home
- Severe breathlessness
- Poor physical function
- Cyanosed
- Severe peripheral oedema
- Impaired consciousness
- On long term oxygen therapy
- Rapid rate of onset

7.11 What are hospital at-home schemes?

Some hospitals in the UK now operate rapid assessment units for patients referred with COPD.[272] These aim to identify those patients that can safely be managed at home with additional nursing and medical input rather than being admitted.[273] They generally take the form of a full assessment of the patient at the hospital by a multidisciplinary team and discharge to the community with appropriate support. This may include additional equipment (e.g. a nebuliser and compressor or an oxygen concentrator), nursing supervision from visiting respiratory nurse specialists, and increased social service input. Patients remain under the care of the hospital consultant but GPs are made aware of the fact that they are receiving home care.

Home care schemes do reduce hospital admissions but the duration of support patients receive at home may be longer than if they had been admitted. Health status is better in patients treated at home,[274] but the schemes are expensive.[275] Most reports on the implementation of such schemes have come from urban areas and they may be more difficult and more expensive to operate in dispersed rural populations.

7.12 What are early discharge schemes?

Early discharge schemes as used within the UK aim to facilitate the early discharge of patients admitted with exacerbations of COPD by providing a package of care at home.[272,276,277] They aim to identify patients in hospital who could be discharged before they have fully recovered by providing increased support in their homes. Assisted discharge schemes do reduce the number of days spent in hospital but the duration of support they receive may be longer than if they had remained in hospital and some will require readmission.

As with home care schemes (see Q. 7.11), health status is better in patients treated at home.[274] but the schemes are expensive[275] and most reports on the implementation of such schemes have come from urban areas.

7.13 Which drugs are used to treat exacerbations?

Drug therapy for exacerbations at home can be summarized as: increased bronchodilators (beta-2 and anticholinergics); antibiotics; oral steroids; diuretics.

■ Increased breathlessness can usually be managed by adding a short-acting beta agonist or anticholinergic bronchodilator, if the patient is not already receiving these, or by increasing the frequency of existing bronchodilator therapy.

■ Most patients can be managed using conventional inhalers but a few benefit from nebulised therapy. Unlike stable COPD, there is little evidence that nebulising a combination of anticholinergic and beta agonist bronchodilators during an exacerbation improves symptoms or the rate of recovery compared with using a beta agonist alone.[278] Most patients requiring a nebuliser can be managed with 2.5 mg salbutamol given 4–6 hourly for 24–48 hours. Some will need it for longer.

■ Antibiotics are widely prescribed but few trials of antibiotic therapy have been placebo controlled, and few have controlled for the effect of steroid administration or have studied sufficient numbers of patients. Meta analyses have suggested a small, and probably clinically insignificant, benefit of antibiotic therapy.[279,280] Patients having frequent exacerbations should be given a reserve course of antibiotics to keep at home so that they may start them without delay.

■ Oral corticosteroids have been shown to speed recovery, shorten inpatient stays and delay the time to the next exacerbation in patients admitted to hospital with exacerbations of COPD. They appear to have similar effects in patients managed in the community[281,282] but are not necessary for the majority of mild exacerbations unless the increased airflow limitation fails to respond to increased bronchodilator therapy or the patient is already on maintenance oral steroid therapy. Most patients requiring steroid therapy respond to 30 mg prednisolone daily for 7–10 days.

■ Patients who develop peripheral oedema at the time of an exacerbation respond to diuretic therapy, but it is important to monitor serum potassium levels, particularly if they are also receiving high dose beta agonist therapy.

Mucolytics are not usually prescribed in the UK or North America. Unlike the evidence regarding their use in stable disease, randomized controlled trials have shown that there is no benefit from adding mucolytic drugs to conventional therapy at times of exacerbations.

In addition to these specific therapies, patients should be encouraged to maintain an adequate fluid intake and to avoid sedative and hypnotic drugs.

Patients with mild exacerbations need not be reviewed unless their symptoms worsen, but those with more severe exacerbations should be reviewed within 48 hours. If they are no better, corticosteroids should be added if these were not prescribed initially and patients should be reviewed again within 48 hours; alternatively referral to hospital should be considered.

7.14 What is the role of nebulised therapy in treating exacerbations?

Nebulisers are frequently used during exacerbations despite the fact that there is conflicting evidence about the comparative efficacy of the same doses of drug given by nebuliser and inhaler. Nebulisers are often preferred because they are easier to administer[283] and because drug deposition is not dependent on inspiratory effort. This may be a justification for their use. There is little evidence that nebulising a combination of anticholinergic and beta agonist bronchodilators during an exacerbation improves symptoms or the rate of recovery compared with using a beta agonist alone.[278]

7.15 How are exacerbations investigated in hospital?

Patients admitted to hospital need an urgent chest radiograph to look principally for evidence of a pneumothorax or pneumonia. Their arterial blood gas tensions will be measured and the inspired oxygen concentration recorded. They should have a full blood count and urea and electrolyte measurements, and an ECG. Sputum should be sent for culture if it looks purulent. Immediate and subsequent hospital investigations in patients with COPD are summarized in *Table 7.1*.

7.16 How are exacerbations managed in hospital?

Drug management of exacerbations in hospital can be summarized as: bronchodilators; controlled oxygen therapy; oral steroids; antibiotics; diuretics; thromboembolus prophylaxis.

■ Bronchodilator therapy is the mainstay of inpatient treatment. Bronchodilators should be given on arrival and at frequent intervals thereafter. There is no evidence that combining beta agonists with anticholinergics is any more effective than either drug alone but in practice combination therapy is often used, particularly for patients with severe exacerbations.

TABLE 7.1 Investigations required in patients admitted to hospital

Timing	Investigation
Immediate	Chest radiograph
	Arterial blood gases
Subsequently	Full blood count
	Urea and electrolytes
	ECG
	Sputum for culture if it looks purulent

■ Many patients are hypoxaemic when admitted and controlled oxygen therapy should be used to achieve a PaO_2 of at least 6.6 kPa without a significant rise in the $PaCO_2$ or the development of significant acidaemia (pH < 7.26). Until the arterial blood gas tensions are known, patients should receive 24% or 28% oxygen via a Venturi mask. Once the blood gas tensions are determined, oxygen therapy should be adjusted accordingly. It is not uncommon to find significant hypercapnia in patients brought in by ambulance as a result of high concentration oxygen therapy during transfer; stabilization with an appropriate FiO_2 often allows the patient to correct this themselves. If the patient is hypercapnic or acidotic the blood gas measurement must be repeated within 1 hour to determine whether the values are stable, improving or deteriorating. If the patient is not hypercapnic the adequacy of oxygenation can be assessed with pulse oximetry.

■ If patients develop respiratory failure, ventilatory support should be considered. It is now recognized that this is best administered non-invasively but where such services are not available patients may require intubation. The outcome of patients requiring intermittent positive pressure ventilation (IPPV) is better than generally thought, particularly by anaesthetists, and misconceptions about the difficulty of weaning patients or about long term survival should not be allowed to affect the decision about intubation. When considering assisted ventilation the patient's previous exercise tolerance and quality of life, and the presence of comorbidities must be considered.

■ Placebo controlled trials have demonstrated that systemic steroid therapy leads to more rapid improvement in FEV_1, shorter hospital stays and delays relapse in patients with exacerbations of COPD.[281,285,286] It has been shown that 2 weeks of treatment is as effective as 8 and oral therapy is as effective as intravenous. Steroids should be discontinued after the acute episode unless the patient has shown a clear response that has not reached a plateau. In this case steroid therapy should be continued until maximum improvement has been achieved, when oral steroids should be withdrawn if possible.

■ Antibiotic use in exacerbations of COPD is controversial but some studies have shown benefits. The BTS COPD guidelines recommend that antibiotics should be given if two of the following three features are present: increased breathlessness, increased sputum volume or increased sputum purulence.[262] It is rarely necessary to give antibiotics intravenously during an exacerbation of COPD.

■ Patients should be given diuretics if the venous pressure is elevated or if there is peripheral or pulmonary oedema.

■ Post mortem studies have shown that pulmonary emboli are common in patients with COPD and unless there are contraindications, immobile patients should receive appropriate prophylaxis.

7.17 What is the role of oral steroids in treating exacerbations of COPD?

Placebo controlled trials have demonstrated that systemic steroid therapy leads to more rapid improvement in FEV_1, shorter hospital stays and delays relapse in both inpatients and outpatients with exacerbations of COPD. [281,285,286] It has been shown that 2 weeks of treatment is as effective as 8 and oral therapy is as effective as intravenous. Whether these data are relevant to patients with milder exacerbations treated at home is not known.

7.18 What is the role of antibiotics in treating exacerbations of COPD?

Antibiotic use in exacerbations of COPD is controversial but some studies have shown benefits. [280] The BTS COPD guidelines recommend that antibiotics should be given if two of the following three features are present: increased breathlessness, increased sputum volume or increased sputum purulence. [284] It is rarely necessary to give antibiotics intravenously during an exacerbation of COPD.

7.19 How should the choice of antibiotic be made?

The bacteria isolated from the lungs of patients with COPD at the time of an exacerbation are usually sensitive to most broad spectrum antibiotics. Amoxicillin is appropriate for patients who are not allergic to penicillins, but cephalosporins, floxacins (provided they are active against *Strep. pneumoniae*) and macrolides are also effective.

PATIENT QUESTIONS

7.20 What is an exacerbation?

Exacerbations are periods when existing symptoms of COPD worsen, medications appear to be less effective or new symptoms develop. Many patients feel that they have a chest infection and indeed some exacerbations are caused by infection, particularly viral infections, but others may be triggered by dusts that are inhaled or by changes in the weather.

7.21 Will I need to go to hospital?

Most exacerbations of COPD can be treated at home. Occasionally admission to hospital is necessary, particularly if the ability of the lungs to maintain adequate oxygen levels in the blood is affected, or if you are unable to look after yourself at home because of the increased symptoms.

7.22 Why do I keep getting chest infections?

The damage that COPD causes in the lungs affects your body's ability to fight off infections and means that when you get a chest infection it will have a greater impact and cause more symptoms than if you did not have COPD.

7.23 How are exacerbations treated?

Exacerbations are usually treated with increased doses of drugs to open up the air tubes (either larger doses or more frequent doses). You may also be advised to take a course of antibiotics, particularly if your sputum has changed to a darker colour, and you may be given a course of steroid tablets which help minimize the effects of the exacerbation.

Oxygen therapy and non-invasive ventilation

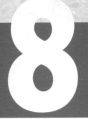

OXYGEN THERAPY

8.1 What forms of oxygen therapy are available?

As the COPD progresses many patients become hypoxaemic. In some the rate of decline in PaO_2 can be as great as 1 kPa per year. Many patients tolerate mild hypoxaemia well, but once the resting PaO_2 falls below 8 kPa patients begin to develop signs of cor pulmonale, principally peripheral oedema. Once this occurs the prognosis is poor and if untreated the 5 year survival is less than 50%.

8.2 What is an oxygen concentrator?

Long term oxygen therapy (LTOT) is usually provided from an oxygen concentrator. These draw ambient air into the unit and pass it through a molecular sieve that adsorbs nitrogen to leave high concentration oxygen that is delivered to the patient.

8.3 What types of oxygen cylinder are available?

The only cylinder officially available on the Drug Tariff in the UK – reimbursed by the Prescriptions Pricing Authority (PPA) – is a 1360 litre 'AF' cylinder, which has a 10 litre water capacity and is filled to 137 bar. These cylinders are 93 cm high and when full weigh 10 kg. A regulator and a flow meter are connected to the cylinder to allow therapy to the patient via tubing and either nasal cannulae or a face mask. The flow meters currently listed on the UK Drug Tariff provide up to 4 l/min only.

Some other cylinders are available on prescription in the UK but are not on the Drug Tariff. Currently the PPA is reimbursing pharmacists for PD, DD and CD cylinders. The PD cylinder is almost 50 cm long and weighs approximately 5 kg. It holds 300 litres of oxygen and requires a flow meter to be attached to it. The PD is still available but is being superseded by the 460 litres lightweight DD cylinder, which is the same size as the PD but weighs just over 4 kg. It holds 460 litres of oxygen and has an integral regulator and flow meter, which can deliver oxygen at 2–4 l/min. Apart from a mask/cannula and tubing, no other equipment needs to be attached to allow delivery of oxygen to the patient.

For patients requiring a flow rate other than 2 or 4 l/min, the CD cylinder (a multiple flow version of the DD) can provide oxygen at 1–15 l/min. Like the DD, the CD holds 460 litres of oxygen and has an integral regulator and flow meter.

8.4 What are the benefits of long term oxygen therapy?

Long term oxygen therapy has been shown to improve survival in patients with COPD who have severe hypoxaemia ($PaO_2 < 8$ kPa).[287,288] Benefits were

---

BOX 8.1 Benefits of long term oxygen therapy

Improved long term survival
Prevention of deterioration in pulmonary hypertension
Reduction of polycythaemia
Improved sleep quality
Increased renal blood flow
Reduction in cardiac arrhythmias

---

seen in patients with a normal or elevated $PaCO_2$, and in patients who had, and had not, had episodes of oedema. The greatest benefits were seen in patients receiving oxygen for 19 hours/day followed by those receiving oxygen for 15 hours/day. Patients receiving oxygen for 12 hours/day had only marginal benefit (*Box 8.1*).

As well as the effects on survival, LTOT leads to less polycythaemia, reduced progression of pulmonary hypertension and improvements in neuropsychological health, but it has only a small beneficial effect on health status. LTOT offers no survival benefit for patients with less severe hypoxia[289] and continuing smoking may negate the benefits of LTOT.[290]

8.5 Which patients require long term oxygen therapy?

Based on the studies described above, current guidelines recommend that LTOT is prescribed for patients with COPD who, *when stable,* have a resting $PaO_2 < 7.3$ kPa, or between 7.3 kPa and 8.0 kPa, and at least one of the following: secondary polycythaemia, nocturnal hypoxia, peripheral oedema or evidence of pulmonary hypertension.[291,292] To get full benefit patients must use LTOT for at least 15 hours/day but patients may get additional benefits from using it for longer periods. CO_2 retention may preclude oxygen therapy in some patients with COPD. Depression of the hypoxic drive to breathe leads to hypercapnia, acidosis and CO_2 narcosis. Some CO_2 retention is tolerable and, depending on the initial value, rises in the $PaCO_2$ of up to 1 kPa may be safe. An arterial stab to measure blood gas tensions is shown in *Figure 8.1*. No patient should receive LTOT without specialist assessment and recommendation (*Table 8.1*).

8.6 How is long term oxygen therapy prescribed?

Within the UK, concentrators can be prescribed by general practitioners in England and Wales and by chest physicians in Scotland. Once a prescription has been written it usually takes 3 or 4 days for the concentrator to be installed. The prescription must specify the oxygen flow rate required, the minimum number of hours per day the patient is to use the oxygen and

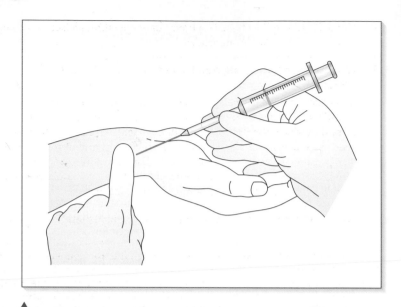

▲

Fig. 8.1 An arterial stab to measure blood gas tensions.

TABLE 8.1 Indicators for referral for long term oxygen therapy assessment

Evidence	Indicator
Severe COPD (FEV$_1$ < 40% predicted normal)	
Hypoxia	Cyanosis
	Polycythaemia (raised haematocrit)
	Confusion or disorientation during acute infection
	Arterial oxygen saturation < 92% on pulse oximeter
	Documented arterial blood gas PaO_2 < 7.3 kPa
Right heart failure	Peripheral oedema (ankle swelling)
	Raised jugular venous pressure
	Weight gain due to fluid retention

whether patients should be supplied with a fixed performance mask (i.e. one that delivers a fixed concentration of oxygen) or nasal cannulae. Nasal cannulae are the most commonly used delivery devices; they are simple to use and are generally comfortable, allowing eating and talking as normal.

Humidification of low flows (1–3 l/min) of oxygen through face masks and nasal cannulae is not recommended.

8.7 What is ambulatory oxygen therapy and what are its benefits?

Ambulatory oxygen therapy provides portable oxygen during exercise and activities of daily living. It may be used as part of continuous oxygen therapy in which case its benefits are those of long term oxygen therapy. When used in isolation the benefits are less clear cut. Ambulatory oxygen therapy can improve exercise tolerance,[293–295] quality of life and compliance with LTOT. Patients derive variable benefits and these cannot be predicted from baseline exercise capacity or lung function impairment.

8.8 Which patients require ambulatory oxygen therapy?

Apart from use as part of long term oxygen therapy, there are no agreed criteria for ambulatory oxygen therapy. However, it is generally agreed that patients who desaturate on exercise (a fall of at least 4% below 90%), who have a ≥10% improvement in exercise capacity and who are motivated to use the oxygen outside the house may benefit from ambulatory oxygen therapy.[292]

■ Ambulatory oxygen therapy in the UK has been traditionally provided from small (230 litre) cylinders. These have a limited capacity, providing only 2 hours at 2 l/min, and cannot be refilled in the patient's home. Oxygen conserving devices, which restrict the flow of oxygen to the inspiratory phase of respiration, have been developed.[296] These can prolong the effective life of the cylinder, but are not prescribable in the UK.

■ Ambulatory oxygen can also be supplied from canisters containing liquid oxygen.[297] These can supply 4 hours of oxygen at 4 l/min. Liquid oxygen is more expensive than gaseous oxygen and is currently unavailable in the UK.

8.9 What are the benefits of short-burst oxygen therapy?

Short-burst oxygen therapy is widely prescribed in the UK[298] and is one of the most expensive therapies used in the National Health Service. Studies have shown variable benefits on exercise capacity[299] and although patients report symptomatic benefit from short-burst therapy after exercise,[300,301] some of this may be due to a cooling effect of the oxygen on the face rather than a correction of hypoxia.

8.10 Which patients require short-burst oxygen therapy?

Intermittent oxygen therapy is commonly prescribed for use by patients who do not meet the criteria for LTOT. The principal indication is breathlessness, often following exertion, which is relieved by oxygen and which is associated with a fall in SaO_2. A recent report from the Royal College of Physicians of London has suggested that short-burst oxygen can be beneficial in patients with severe COPD whose episodic breathlessness is not relieved by other treatments.[292]

8.11 Are there any hazards of oxygen therapy?

Fire and explosion are real dangers and there have been many reports of patients starting fires, usually by lighting a cigarette whilst wearing nasal cannulae.[302] Patients and their families and carers must be warned not to smoke in the vicinity of the oxygen.

VENTILATION

8.12 What is non-invasive ventilation?

Non-invasive ventilation is a method of providing ventilatory support that does not require the placement of an endotracheal tube. In the absence of other organ system failure, and provided that the patient does not have large volumes of secretions and is able to cooperate, non-invasive ventilation (NIV) is now considered the treatment of choice for patients with hypercapnic respiratory failure.[303] This is usually delivered via a mask that covers the nose, but occasionally a full face mask covering the nose and the mouth is required. Patients treated with NIV are less likely to need intubation, and mortality rates are reduced.[304]

NIV may be used as a holding measure (to assist ventilation in patients at an earlier stage than that at which intubation would be considered); as a trial (with a view to intubation if it fails); or as the ceiling of treatment in patients who are not candidates for intubation. The outcome of patients who remain acidotic (pH < 7.30) after initial treatment is less good and these patients are best managed in a high dependency setting by experienced clinicians.

8.13 What are the benefits of non-invasive ventilation in COPD?

Patients treated with NIV are less likely to need intubation, and mortality rates are reduced.[304] NIV can be used intermittently and this has obvious

---

BOX 8.2 Contraindications to non-invasive ventilation

■ Coma or confusion
■ Inability to protect the airway
■ Severe acidosis at presentation
■ Copious respiratory secretions
■ Significant comorbidity
■ Vomiting
■ Obstructed bowel
■ Haemodynamic instability
■ Radiological evidence of consolidation
■ Orofacial abnormalities that interfere with the mask/face interface

---

advantages during weaning. Patients are usually able to eat and drink when using NIV and they can communicate with staff and visitors.

8.14 What are the contraindications to non-invasive ventilation?

There are relatively few contraindications to the use of non-invasive ventilation (NIV) in COPD. The principal ones are multiorgan system failure, the inability to cooperate with the treatment or the inability to protect the airway (*Box 8.2*). It is difficult to clear excessive volumes of mucus when using NIV and patients with a lot of sputum may therefore be unable to cope with this method of ventilatory support.

8.15 Where can non-invasive ventilation be performed?

NIV may be performed in an intensive therapy unit (ITU) or on a general ward.[305] In the UK there is an increasing trend to perform NIV in respiratory high dependency units attached to or part of respiratory wards. This allows the development of nursing and medical expertise.

8.16 What is the role of ITU in patients with COPD?

It is commonly believed that patients admitted to intensive therapy units (ITU) because of an exacerbation of COPD have a poor prognosis. In fact, recent studies have shown that significant survival rates can be achieved even when there is marked physiological derangement.[306,307] The introduction of non-invasive ventilation (NIV) has meant that many patients with ventilatory failure secondary to an exacerbation of COPD (*see Q. 7.16*) can be managed outside the ITU, but even so mortality rates in those patients who need more intensive support are as good as in studies prior to the introduction of NIV.[307]

Intubation and ventilation may be necessary in patients who are unable to cooperate with NIV or protect their airways, those who are producing large volumes of sputum, those who remain hypoxic or acidotic despite NIV, and those who develop signs of systemic sepsis or multiorgan system failure. ITU treatment is associated with high emotional stress on patients and their families and it may not be appropriate in those with a poor prognosis. FEV_1 is a poor indicator of prognosis,[308] but premorbid activity levels are good indicators, with higher mortality in patients who are housebound.[308,309]

 PATIENT QUESTIONS

8.17 Why do some patients need oxygen?

As COPD progresses the level of oxygen in the blood falls. In some patients this fall puts a strain on the heart and unless treated with oxygen their condition rapidly worsens. These patients need to breathe oxygen for at least 16 hours each day. In patients with less severe disease oxygen levels sometimes fall during exertion and some of these patients are able to do more if they breathe oxygen during exertion. All patients being considered for oxygen therapy need careful assessment as oxygen can be harmful to some patients.

8.18 How can I tell if I need oxygen?

In general patients cannot tell if they need oxygen. If you are becoming more breathless when performing simple tasks such as washing or dressing you may need oxygen and your doctor will be able to assess this. If your doctor thinks you may need oxygen, a visit to the hospital to have the oxygen levels in your blood measured will probably be arranged.

8.19 Can machines be used to help my breathing?

Machines are now available which can help patients breathe during exacerbations of their COPD. They help to get the air down into the lungs and can also help the lungs empty more efficiently. To use them, the patient must wear a tightly fitting mask which covers either just their nose or their nose and their mouth. These machines are often needed only for short periods whilst the exacerbation responds to treatment. As the patient's breathing improves, the machine can be used intermittently, helping with breathing when the patient gets tired. Used in this way these machines have helped many patients avoid the need for a tube in their throat and the need for treatment on an intensive therapy unit.

A few people with COPD need to use such machines at home during periods when they are stable. This is uncommon, is not usually necessary and requires considerable back-up from a hospital.

Pulmonary rehabilitation and non-pharmacological management of COPD

9

PULMONARY REHABILITATION

9.1 What is pulmonary rehabilitation?

Pulmonary rehabilitation is an increasingly popular and effective option for patients with moderate to severe COPD. Rehabilitation aims to prevent deconditioning and allow the patient to cope with the disease. Most programmes are hospital based and comprise individualized exercise programmes (*Fig. 9.1*) and educational talks, but a major component is the sharing of experiences amongst participants and their spouses.

Programmes are widely available in North America and Europe, but availability is still limited in the UK. The detailed content of the programmes varies considerably but this seems to have little effect on outcome[310] (*Box 9.1*).

There are no specific referral criteria but patients must be sufficiently mobile and motivated to attend the programme.[311]

9.2 Where are pulmonary rehabilitation programmes run?

In the UK most programmes are based in secondary care. These are effective but may suffer from a high drop-out rate and patients may be deterred from attending by the frequent journeys to the hospital.[312]

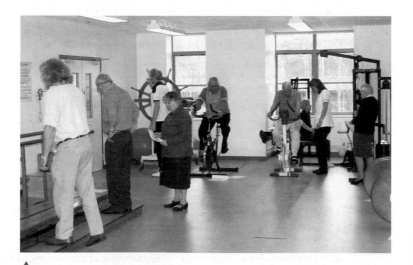

▲
Fig. 9.1 Patients undergoing pulmonary rehabilitation.

BOX 9.1   Essential components of pulmonary rehabilitation programmes

■ Exercise training
■ Education about:
   — the disease and its management
   — benefits and financial support available
   — travel
■ Psychological and behavioural interventions
■ Outcome assessment

Rehabilitation programmes for use at home have also been developed. These may be less effective because patients do not perform the prescribed exercises and miss the group therapy aspects of hospital-based programmes. There is now growing interest in running programmes in primary care.[313]

9.3   What are the benefits of pulmonary rehabilitation?

Pulmonary rehabilitation can reduce symptoms, increase mobility, improve quality of life[310,314,315] and may also reduce hospital readmission rates. Benefits of pulmonary rehabilitation programmes include:

■ increased exercise capacity
■ better health status
■ reduced primary care consultation rates
■ reduced hospital admissions.

9.4   How widely available is pulmonary rehabilitation?

Pulmonary rehabilitation courses are becoming widely available, but it is estimated that only just over half of all hospitals in the UK offer a programme. The British Lung Foundation can provide up to date information about the availability of programmes in the UK (*see Ch. 14*).

9.5   What can I do if a pulmonary rehabilitation programme is not available?

Even if a formal pulmonary rehabilitation programme is not available locally patients can help themselves by undertaking exercise at home. They should be advised to do some exercise each day and to set realistic goals (*Box 9.2*).

BOX 9.2 Advice about exercise for patients if a rehabilitation programme is not available locally

■ Discuss plans with your general practitioner/primary care physician
■ Start small
■ Walk every day
■ Pace yourself
■ Start during the spring and summer
■ Exercise consistently and set realistic goals
■ Educate yourself:
— ask for advice
— read information leaflets, e.g. from the British Lung Foundation
— write down questions for your general practitioner/primary care physician or practice nurse
■ Keep exercising during winter
■ Keep going even during bad times
■ Consider joining a support organization, e.g. 'Breathe Easy' (*see Appendix*)

NUTRITION

9.6 Why do patients with COPD lose weight?

Many patients with COPD lose weight as a consequence of decreased food intake as a result of breathlessness, altered absorption as a result of hypoxia and increased resting energy expenditure as a result of the increased work of breathing.[316] The mechanisms of this remain unclear but probably relate to systemic effects of cytokines, particularly tumour necrosis factor alpha (TNF-α).[317]

9.7 What is the significance of a low body mass index?

Many patients with COPD lose weight as a consequence of decreased food intake as a result of breathlessness, altered absorption as a result of hypoxia and increased resting energy expenditure as a result of the increased work of breathing.[316] Patients who are underweight have an increased mortality and this can be reduced by appropriate nutritional support.[318] Loss of muscle mass is an independent predictor of outcome in COPD and is an area infrequently addressed by therapy.[318]

9.8   Does nutritional supplementation improve outcomes in COPD?

If patients have a low body mass index, correction of this using dietary supplementation has been shown to improve survival. There are no benefits in patients who are not underweight.

9.9   Are there certain foods to avoid?

There are no specific foods to avoid in COPD. Some patients may benefit from avoiding gas-forming vegetables such as beans, cabbage and peppers which can lead to abdominal distension and diaphragmatic splinting, leading to worsening breathlessness. Patients who produce large amounts of mucus often seem to benefit by reducing or eliminating dairy produce from their diets.

9.10   What should patients with COPD be advised about their diet?

Dieticians recommend that patients maintain an adequate fluid intake, have an adequate intake of calories, protein, calcium, and potassium. Patients with more advanced disease often benefit from eating small portions frequently as they can feel more breathless after large meals, probably as a result of diaphragmatic splinting. For the same reasons some patients may benefit from avoiding gas-forming vegetables such as beans, cabbage and peppers. Patients who produce large amounts of mucus often seem to benefit by reducing or eliminating dairy produce from their diets.

VACCINATION

9.11   Should patients with COPD receive an annual influenza vaccine?

Although there have been no studies specifically in patients with COPD, vaccination of patients with chronic respiratory disease against influenza has been shown to reduce hospital attendance and admission rates and death rates from influenza.[319–321] Annual influenza vaccination is recommended for all patients with COPD.[322,323]

9.12   Should patients with COPD receive a pneumococcal vaccine?

It is now also common to vaccinate patients against the pneumococcus using the polyvalent capsular polysaccharide vaccine.[324] This has been shown to reduce the incidence of invasive pneumococcal disease in patients with chronic lung disease[325] and to be cost effective.[319]

TRAVEL

9.13 Can patients with COPD fly?

Many patients with COPD continue to want to travel. Travel within the UK is usually not a problem and oxygen concentrators can be transported in cars. Flying may present more difficulties as the reduced cabin pressure may lead to significant hypoxia. Aircraft cabins are not usually pressurized to sea level and patients with compensated COPD at sea level may experience significant hypoxaemia when flying. Patients may become breathless, wheezy or develop chest pain and on long flights right heart failure may develop. Patients should be advised to ensure that they carry their inhalers in their hand luggage.

Procedures for requesting in-flight oxygen and costs differ between airlines but most require medical authorization and at least 48 hours' notice prior to departure.[326] Patients should check with the airline at the time of booking.

9.14 Which patients with COPD need oxygen during flight?

The best predictor of the need for in-flight oxygen is the PaO_2 on the ground. Criteria for assessing the need for in-flight oxygen are shown in *Table 9.1*.[327]

Patients on long term oxygen therapy need in-flight oxygen and should make their own provision for oxygen during waiting periods at airports.

TABLE 9.1 Assessing need for in-flight oxygen

Oxygen saturation	Oxygen requirement
$SpO_2 > 95\%$	Oxygen not required in flight
SpO_2 92–95%:	
No additional risk factor	Oxygen not required in flight
Hypercapnia, ventilatory support, recent exacerbation, cardiac disease, cerebrovascular disease	Need a formal assessment of need for in-flight oxygen
$SpO_2 < 92\%$	Need in-flight oxygen

PATIENT QUESTIONS

9.15   Should I try to exercise?

Regular exercise within the limitations imposed by breathlessness maintains fitness and reduces disability. Even patients who have not been used to taking any exercise can benefit from graded exercises, particularly when part of a pulmonary rehabilitation programme.

9.16   What is pulmonary rehabilitation?

Pulmonary rehabilitation is an effective way of improving patients' breathing, their ability to perform everyday tasks and their ability to cope with their illness. Rehabilitation aims to help patients regain some of their fitness by undertaking gentle graded exercises under supervision. It also provides an opportunity to share experiences of coping with the disease with other patients and provides education to help patients understand their disease, its treatments and ways of coping. Most programmes are hospital based but increasingly pulmonary rehabilitation courses are being run in the community and this has a number of advantages. The exercise sessions are usually backed up by at least one session of exercise at home and some patients move on to specific exercise programmes at local sports centres at the end of the programme.

9.17   Should I be on a special diet?

There is no evidence that specific diets are beneficial for patients with COPD, but it is important that patients are not overweight as this may worsen their breathlessness on exertion. Some patients with advanced disease lose weight as part of the illness and this may lead to weakness of the chest muscles. These patients need to maintain an adequate calorie intake. Patients who produce significant amounts of sputum observe that the amount of sputum is reduced and it is easier to cough it up if they reduce the amount of dairy produce in their diet. The reason for this is not known.

9.18   Why do I keep losing weight?

Because of the damage to the lungs patients with COPD have to work harder to breathe and this extra effort burns up calories. COPD also affects other parts of the body in ways that cause weight loss. These effects together with the fact that many patients find eating large meals makes them more breathless explain the weight loss in most patients. Occasionally weight loss is due to other more serious causes and if the weight loss is new or becomes more rapid you should consult you doctor.

9.19   Should I have a flu vaccination?

It is a good idea for all patients with COPD to have an annual influenza vaccination unless they have had a previous allergic reaction to the vaccine.

9.20   Can I still go on holiday?

Many patients with COPD continue to travel. Some patients may need to arrange for oxygen to be available on aircraft and may need wheelchair assistance at airports or train stations. Patients should always ensure that they take adequate supplies of all their medications with them and that they have appropriate insurance.

9.21   How can I arrange to have oxygen during a flight?

The procedures for requesting in-flight oxygen and costs differ between airlines. You should check on the exact procedure with the airline at the time of booking. It is important to remember that airlines generally require at least 48 hours' notice prior to departure in order to make sure the oxygen is put on the flight. Most airlines require medical authorization and this can be provided by your doctor.

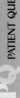

Surgical management of COPD

10

PQ PATIENT QUESTIONS

10.1 Are any surgical treatments available?

Over the last 50 years many surgical interventions to improve breathlessness in patients with COPD have been tried. In general these have been ineffective and have carried high mortality.[328] During the past 15 years lung transplantation has been used successfully in COPD but availability of organs has seriously limited its application in the UK. Recently, surgery to remove functionless areas of lung in patients with COPD has also been shown to have benefits. This is known as lung volume reduction surgery (LVRS) and works by improving the mechanics of breathing by reducing thoracic volumes.

10.2 What is bullectomy?

Bullectomy is the surgical excision of single large bullae occupying at least one-third of a hemithorax. It has been used for many years[329] and the two main indications are pneumothorax or chronic disabling breathlessness. The evidence of its effectiveness on breathlessness is limited but the best results appear to be in patients with demonstrable compression of normal lung tissue.[330] This is now best visualized on CT scanning. Operative mortality rates ranging from 0 to 8% have been reported.[330] The procedure can be complicated by persistent air leaks and in order to overcome this intracavity drainage combined with instillation of a sclerosant has been developed.[331]

10.3 What is lung volume reduction surgery?

Lung volume reduction surgery (LVRS) is surgery designed to remove functionless areas of lung in patients with COPD. It works by improving the mechanics of breathing by reducing thoracic volumes. It was initially used as a palliative procedure in patients awaiting lung transplantation but it has become a procedure in its own right and around the world thousands of patients have now undergone this operation successfully.

10.4 Which patients are suitable for lung volume reduction surgery?

Patient selection for lung volume reduction surgery is crucial. The indications for LVRS (*Box 10.1*) are severe physiological impairment ($FEV_1 < 35\%$), marked hyperinflation and severe disability despite maximal medical therapy. Patients who have heterogenous disease on CT are more suitable for LVRS. Hypercapnia ($PaCO_2 > 55$ mmHg) or a diffusing capacity less than 20% predicted are contraindications.[332]

BOX 10.1 Indications for lung volume reduction surgery

- Severe airflow limitation ($FEV_1 < 35\%$)
- Hyperinflation
- Severe disability
- Heterogenous disease on CT scan

10.5 What are the benefits and risks of lung volume reduction surgery?

Lung volume reduction surgery produces clinically and statistically significant improvements in FEV_1, shuttle walking distance and quality of life,[333] but does not appear to affect mortality.

10.6 Can lung transplantation be used in COPD?

Single or bilateral lung transplantation is only indicated in COPD if the patient's condition has deteriorated to the point that they are severely limited and their estimated life expectancy is short. Older patients have a significantly higher operative mortality and a worse long term survival than younger patients[334] and most units will not transplant patients aged over 65.

10.7 Which patients are suitable for lung transplantation?

 Indications for transplantation are shown in *Box 10.2.* Symptomatic osteoporosis is a relative contraindication and patients with a high or a low body mass index require either nutritional support or weight loss prior to transplantation. Use of low dose (< 20 mg/day prednisolone) is not now considered a contraindication to transplantation.[335]

10.8 What are the benefits and risks of lung transplantation?

Postoperatively there are improvements in lung function, PaO_2, walking distance and health status, but overall transplants do not appear to improve long term survival. The current 5 year survival figures are around 50%[336–338] (*see also Ch. 14*).

BOX 10.2 Indications for single lung transplantation

- Severe airflow limitation ($FEV_1 < 25\%$)
- Respiratory failure ($PaCO_2 > 7.3$ kPa)
- Severe disability
- Progressive deterioration
- Pulmonary hypertension

PATIENT QUESTIONS

10.9 Could an operation help me?

Operations can help a very small minority of patients with COPD who have areas of badly affected lung which are either squashing other areas of better lung and stopping them working properly or making it difficult for the chest muscles to work efficiently. Very occasionally an operation to transplant a healthy lung into patients with COPD can be performed.

10.10 Could I have a lung transplant?

Lung transplants in COPD have been performed but the operation carries a substantial mortality and relatively few lungs become available for transplantation. The risks of the operation rise significantly with increasing age and for this reason transplants are not usually performed beyond the age of 65. Because of the risks of the operation it is not usually performed until the symptoms and expected survival without an operation are sufficient to justify the risks. This generally means that the patient is wheelchair bound and oxygen dependent.

New treatments

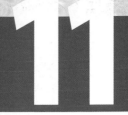

11.1 What types of new treatment are being developed for COPD?

A number of anti-inflammatory drugs and specific mediator antagonists are in development[339] and if they prove effective they may both improve symptoms and prevent or slow disease progression.

Drugs that reduce mucus secretion or improve mucociliary clearance are also in development. Some block the inflammatory signals that lead to increased mucus secretion whilst others inhibit mucin secretion. Intriguingly, macrolide antibiotics have been shown act in this way[340] and this may partially explain their actions in treating exacerbations.

11.2 What are PDE4 inhibitors?

PDE4 inhibitors are drugs which inhibit phosphodiesterase type 4 (PDE4). They can cause bronchodilatation and inhibit neutrophilic inflammation. They reduce breathlessness, improve health status and may also reduce exacerbations, but their use may be limited by the fact that a significant proportion of patients develop transient gastrointestinal side-effects.[341]

 PATIENT QUESTIONS

11.3 Is research being carried out into new treatments for COPD?

Enormous efforts are being devoted to developing new and more effective treatments for COPD. These are being backed up by research to understand why COPD develops and which cells and chemical messengers are involved in its progression. There is every reason to expect that effective new treatments will be developed over the next 10–15 years.

11.4 How can I find out about new treatments?

Your doctor may be aware of new treatments for COPD that are in the final stages of development or that have just become available. Patient support groups such as the British Lung Foundation (*see Ch. 14*) may also have information. Newspapers and on-line news services may also carry articles about new research or new treatments.

PATIENT QUESTIONS

Palliative care

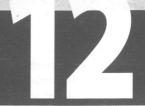

12.1 What information do patients with advanced COPD need to help them cope with the future?

Patients need to be given honest and clear information about the progressive nature of COPD and the treatments that are available to manage advanced disease, including mechanical ventilation, intubation and palliative care strategies. Many patients feel that they have not received enough information about the prognosis and future management.[342] In contrast, most patients stated that they want broad indications of prognosis but did not want detailed information that they perceived would be distressing.[342] There is often a perception that patients have received mixed messages from different health professionals.

Many physicians are reluctant to discuss intubation and ventilation with patients[343] and patients often end up being admitted with a severe exacerbation without these issues having been discussed. They are then too ill to be able to express their wishes, resulting in decisions being made by physicians, family members or surrogates.

As well as information about their disease, patients need information about what financial and social support is available.[344]

12.2 What is the role of palliative care services?

Once it is clear that a patient is in the terminal stages of their disease, adequate symptom palliation is essential. The emphasis of care is often on preventing hospitalization, but these efforts may neglect day to day symptoms with the result that patients live with high levels of symptoms.[344] Non-pharmacological approaches, including counselling, breathing retraining, relaxation and teaching of coping strategies can help.[345] Patients also need support in the community from health and social services.[344]

12.3 How can the symptoms of end stage COPD be palliated?

Anxiety can be controlled using buspirone (which does not suppress respiration[346]) or benzodiazepines. If rapid control is required, 0.5–2 mg lorazepam sublingually is effective. Diazepam 5–10 mg daily is appropriate to maintain control.

Breathlessness can be controlled using opiates (e.g. 2.5 mg diamorphine every 4 hours). If patients are unable to swallow, drug treatment can be continued using a subcutaneous infusion administered using a syringe driver. Pharmacological approaches to palliative care are summarized in *Box 12.1*.

Non-pharmacological approaches, including counselling, breathing retraining, relaxation and teaching of coping strategies can help.[345]

BOX 12.1 Drug therapy in palliative care

■ Benzodiazepines to control anxiety
■ Opiates to control breathlessness
■ Consider continuous subcutaneous infusion therapy

12.4 Should patients be encouraged to make advance directives?

Advance directives or living wills are a logical extension of the involvement of patients in decisions about their care.[347] Many patients have strong views about issues such as whether they would want to receive ventilatory support or be resuscitated in the event of a cardiac or respiratory arrest and it is very useful to have these wishes recorded. It is obviously essential that patients are fully informed of the practicalities and benefits of such treatments, as there are often misconceptions, and they must be considered competent to make a decision. Many patients feel that this is an area that is not discussed by their doctors.[348] It is also important to remember that patients' attitude to what comprises satisfactory quality of life changes with advancing disease.

 PATIENT QUESTIONS

12.5 Will I suffer as my COPD gets worse?

The symptoms of advanced COPD are similar to those of milder disease, but breathlessness often develops after undertaking simpler tasks. Modern treatment is able to relieve these symptoms even though it cannot cure COPD.

12.6 Will my COPD kill me?

COPD is the cause of death in some patients, usually in association with a severe chest infection. Many patients with COPD die of other causes that affect the general population, although there is obviously an increased risk of death from smoking related causes such as heart disease, strokes and cancer.

12.7 What can I do to make sure the doctors treat me in the way that I want?

Many patients with serious long term disease now let their doctors know how they would want to be treated in particular circumstances by writing these views down. These documents are sometimes known as advance directives or living wills. If you do have strong views about how you want to be treated you should discuss these with your doctors to make sure you and they understand the effects of these views. It is also important to be sure that you are aware fully aware of what these treatments involve.

Practice organization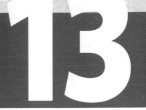

13.1 What is the role of practice nurses?

It is likely that nurses such as those attached to general practices within the UK will be able to contribute to the management of patients with COPD but their roles are still being defined and many still have no formal training in COPD. There may be some overlap with service based in secondary care such as outreach nursing, hospital at-home and assisted discharge schemes, as well as involvement in community-based pulmonary rehabilitation programmes.

- Nurse-run COPD clinics in primary care are likely to become increasingly important in the management of COPD in the community. Practice nurses have shown great enthusiasm for acquiring the knowledge and skills to differentiate asthma from COPD and many are trained to perform spirometry.
- Nurse-facilitated self-management plans for COPD have been piloted,[349] and nurse-led clinics have been shown to reduce the need for general practitioner/primary care physician (GP/PCP) interventions.[350]
- Nurses have more time available to provide patients with education about their disease and the use of medication and nurses are well placed to facilitate smoking cessation (*see Ch. 14*).
- If nurses are to fulfil these roles safely, however, adequate training is essential.[351]

13.2 Is there a role for COPD clinics?

As with asthma, the organization of care is vitally important. Although structured care for patients with COPD is only just being introduced there is evidence that it reduces emergency consultations, improves patients' understanding of their disease and their ability to self-manage, and gives an opportunity to rationalize therapy and identify complications.

13.3 What education should be provided for patients with COPD?

All published guidelines emphasize the importance of providing education for patients with COPD but there have been very few studies on its effect in isolation or exactly what information is needed. It has been shown that the effects of education in patients with COPD differ significantly from the effects in asthma.[352]

- Group sessions, backed up by written information, dealing with the nature of the lung abnormalities, the effects of medication,

---

BOX 13.1 Topics that may need covering in patient education sessions (based on Pulmonary rehabilitation[354])

■ Disease background (anatomy, physiology, pathology and pharmacology, including oxygen therapy and vaccination)
■ Dyspnoea/symptom management, including chest clearance techniques
■ Smoking cessation
■ Energy conservation/pacing
■ Nutritional advice
■ Managing travel
■ Benefits system and disabled parking badges
■ Advance directives
■ Anxiety management
■ Goal setting and rewards
■ Relaxation
■ Loving relationships/sexuality
■ Exacerbation management (including when to seek help, self-management and decision making, coping with setbacks and relapses)
■ Home care support
■ The benefits of physical exercise
■ Support groups

---

and including a discussion of the symptoms that occur, the early signs of an exacerbation and fears about side-effects of therapy have been shown to reduce GP/PCP visits and probably improve quality of life, but their effects on patients' symptoms was not reported.[352]

■ Education must be tailored to patients' needs (*see Box 13.1*). Some patients do not want to know about aspects of their disease, particularly prognosis, and education can increase anxiety levels.[353]

13.4 Do self-management plans improve outcomes in COPD?

Given the similarities between COPD and asthma management, it has been suggested that patients with COPD could also benefit from having self-management plans. There are, however, important differences such as the lack of response to inhaled steroids and the greater reliance on regular bronchodilator therapy that make COPD self-management plans more difficult to agree and implement. Nevertheless, plans that include recommendations on an early response to exacerbations, as well as guidance on taking regular exercise, healthy eating and scheduling activities according to levels of symptoms have been developed.[349,355] These plans increase oral steroid use and reduce rescue medication use but do not appear to reduce hospitalization rates. They may improve patients' quality of life, but the effects on daily symptoms are less clear.

13.5 Does visiting patients at home on a regular basis improve outcomes in COPD?

A number of studies have looked at the effects of visiting patients at home on a regular basis.[356–359] These services are usually run by nurses and are known as outreach nursing. In patients with milder disease such services may reduce mortality and may improve health related quality of life, although the effects are small.[360] Outreach nursing does not appear to reduce mortality and hospital admissions or improve quality of life in patients with more severe disease.[360]

PATIENT QUESTIONS

13.6 Do I need to attend the surgery regularly?

Because COPD is a progressive disease it is sensible to have your symptoms assessed and lung function checked once a year, but provided you are keeping well in between there is no evidence that regular check ups are necessary. Obviously you should contact the surgery if there is any significant or sustained change in your symptoms. The surgery will probably also contact you in the autumn to ask you to have an annual influenza vaccination.

13.7 Can I do anything to monitor the disease myself?

Being aware of how much you feel able to do each day and how bad your symptoms are compared to normal is the best way to monitor your disease. By being aware of increased breathlessness or changes in the amount or colour of sputum you produce, you may be able to detect an exacerbation before it gets too bad. Noting situations that make your breathing worse can also be helpful. It is also important to check your weight and make sure that you are eating adequate amounts of healthy foods.

Sources of further information

14

SOURCES OF FURTHER INFORMATION

14.1 Which professional societies produce information about COPD?

The British Thoracic Society, through its COPD Consortium, produces a range of materials to help healthcare professionals manage patients with COPD. They have produced brief summaries of the 1997 guidelines and the position statement on pulmonary rehabilitation as well as a booklet on performing spirometry in practice and a series of booklets on managing patients with COPD in primary care. The Consortium's publications can be accessed via the BTS web site (www.brit-thoracic.org.uk).

14.2 Which patient support organizations and charities produce information about COPD?

In the UK the British Lung Foundation (BLF) produces a range of leaflets about lung disease and COPD. Through their 'Breathe Easy' clubs patients can also meet other patients with COPD and learn more about this and other respiratory conditions from regular educational meetings. The BLF can be contacted via their web site (www.lunguk.org). Information is also available from the American Lung Association (www.lungusa.org) and the Canadian Lung Foundation (www.lung.ca/copd/). Information specifically about alpha-1 antitrypsin deficiency is available from Alpha one (www.alpha1.org).

14.3 Which organizations provide training in managing patients with COPD?

In the UK training for nurses involved in the management of COPD is provided by a number of organizations including the National Respiratory Training Centre (www.nartc.org.uk) and the Respiratory Education and Training Centres (RETC) (www.respiratoryetc.com). Many hospitals also provide local updates on COPD management.

14.4 Which organizations provide information about smoking cessation?

Both Action on Smoking and Health (ASH) (www.ash.org.uk) and Quit (www.quit.org) are UK-based charities that provide information about stopping smoking. Information about the National Health Service (NHS) smoking cessation services is also available from the NHS smoking cessation website (www.doh.gov.uk/tobacco/cessation.htm). Internationally, information is available from the WHO tobacco free initiative (www5.who.int/tobacco/) and the USA tobacco cessation guideline (www.surgeongeneral.gov/tobacco/).

14.5   Which companies provide information about COPD?

Many of the pharmaceutical and medical equipment manufacturers provide information about their products and respiratory diseases in general as well as specific information about COPD. They can often be contacted via their web sites:

- 3M (www.3m.com/us/healthcare/pharma)
- AstraZeneca (www.astrazeneca.com)
- BOC Group (www.boc.com)
- Boehringer Ingelheim (www.boehringer-ingelheim.com)
- Clement Clarke (www.clement-clarke.com)
- Ferraris (www.ferrarismedical.com)
- GlaxoSmithKline (www.gsk.com)
- Micro Medical (www.micromedical.co.uk)
- Napp (www.napp.co.uk)
- Novartis (www.novatis.com)
- Vitalograph (www.vitalograph.co.uk)

 PATIENT QUESTIONS

14.6   How can I learn more about COPD?

A number of leaflets and booklets have been produced to help you understand more about COPD and your lungs. Your doctor or practice nurse may have some of these. You can also contact the British Lung Foundation (www.lunguk.org or 020 7831 5831). Information is also available from the American Lung Association (www.lungusa.org) and the Canadian Lung Foundation (www.lung.ca/copd/). Information specifically about alpha-1 antitrypsin deficiency is available from Alpha one (www.alpha1.org).

OTHER SOURCES OF INFORMATION

- ASH Scotland (www.ashscotland.org.uk)
- Australian Lung Foundation (www.lungnet.org.au/)
- AZ-Air (www.az-air.com)
- BMJ collected articles on COPD
  (http://bmj.com/cgi/collection/chronic_obstructive_airways)
- Chest net (www.chestnet.net)
- Colorado HealthSite
  (www.coloradohealthsite.org/COPD/copd_main.html)
- COPDprofessional (www.copdprofessional.hmg.com)
- General Practice Airways group (www.gpiag.org)
- GOLD COPD guidelines for Palm OS
  (http://hin.nhlbi.nih.gov/copd.htm)
- GOLD Initiative (www.goldcopd.com)
- Health Education Board for Scotland (HEBS) web site (for smoking
  cessation guidelines and patient information)
  (www.hebs.co.uk/topics/smoking/index.htm; www.hebs.com/tobacco/)
- International Society for Heart and Lung Transplantation
  (www.ishlt.org)
- Lung and Asthma Information Agency
  (www.sghms.ac.uk/laia/laiaadmin.htm), National Asthma Campaign
  (www.asthma.org.uk)
- Mayo Clinic (www.mayo.edu)
- MedlinePlus COPD resources
  (www.nlm.nih.gov/medlineplus/copdchronicobstructivepulmonarydise
  ase.html)

REFERENCES

Definition and epidemiology

1. COPD Guidelines Group of the Standards of Care Committee of the BTS. BTS guidelines for the management of chronic obstructive pulmonary disease. Thorax 1997;52(Suppl 5):S1–28.

2. Pauwels RA, Buist AS, Calverley PM, Jenkins CR, Hurd SS. Global strategy for the diagnosis, management, and prevention of chronic obstructive pulmonary disease. NHLBI/WHO Global Initiative for Chronic Obstructive Lung Disease (GOLD) Workshop summary. Am J Respir Crit Care Med 2001;163(5):1256–1276.

3. Doll R, Peto R, Wheatley K, Gray R, Sutherland I. Mortality in relation to smoking: 40 years' observations on male British doctors. BMJ 1994;309(6959):901–911.

4. Coggon D, Newman Taylor A. Coal mining and chronic obstructive pulmonary disease: a review of the evidence. Thorax 1998;53(5):398–407.

5. Pride NB, Connellan SJ. Chronic bronchitis in non-smokers. Introductory review. Eur J Respir Dis Suppl 1982;118:9–14.

6. Hendrick DJ. Occupational and chronic obstructive pulmonary disease (COPD). Thorax 1996;51(9):947–955.

7. Barker DJ, Godfrey KM, Fall C, Osmond C, Winter PD, Shaheen SO. Relation of birth weight and childhood respiratory infection to adult lung function and death from chronic obstructive airways disease. BMJ 1991;303(6804):671–675.

8. Shaheen S, Barker DJ. Early lung growth and chronic airflow obstruction. Thorax 1994;49(6):533–536.

9. Shahar E, Folsom AR, Melnick SL, et al. Dietary n-3 polyunsaturated fatty acids and smoking-related chronic obstructive pulmonary disease. Atherosclerosis Risk in Communities Study Investigators. N Engl J Med 1994;331(4):228–233.

10. Britton JR, Pavord ID, Richards KA, et al. Dietary antioxidant vitamin intake and lung function in the general population. Am J Respir Crit Care Med 1995;151(5):1383–1387.

11. Sluiter HJ, Koeter GH, de Monchy JG, Postma DS, de Vries K, Orie NG. The Dutch hypothesis (chronic non-specific lung disease) revisited. Eur Respir J 1991;4(4):479–489.

12. Fletcher C, Peto R, Tinker C, Speizer F. The natural history of chronic bronchitis and emphysema. An 8 year study of working men. Oxford: Oxford University Press; 1976.

13. Hunninghake GW, Crystal R. Cigarette smoking and lung destruction: accumulation of neutrophils in the lungs of cigarette smokers. Am Rev Respir Dis 1983;128:833–838.

14. Stratton K, Shetty P, Wallace R, Bondurant S, eds. Clearing the smoke: assessing the science base for tobacco harm reduction. Washington, DC: National Academy Press; 2001.

15. Rahman I, MacNee W. Role of oxidants/antioxidants in smoking-induced lung diseases. Free Radic Biol Med 1996;21(5):669–681.

16. Morrison D, Rahman I, Lannan S, MacNee W. Epithelial permeability, inflammation, and oxidant stress in the

air spaces of smokers. Am J Respir Crit Care Med 1999;159(2):473–479.

17. Hinman LM, Stevens CA, Matthay RA, Gee JB. Elastase and lysozyme activities in human alveolar macrophages: effects of cigarette smoking. Am Rev Respir Dis 1980;116:263–271.

18. Hautamaki RD, Kobayashi D, Senior RM, Shapiro SD. Requirement for macrophage elastase for cigarette smoke-induced emphysema in mice. Science 1997;277:2002–2004.

19. Janoff A, Carp H. Possible mechanisms of emphysema in smokers: cigarette smoke condensate suppresses protease inhibition in vitro. Am Rev Respir Dis 1977;116(1):65–72.

20. Totti N, 3rd, McCusker KT, Campbell EJ, Griffin GL, Senior RM. Nicotine is chemotactic for neutrophils and enhances neutrophil responsiveness to chemotactic peptides. Science 1984;223(4632):169–171.

21. Beck GJ, Doyle CA, Schachter EN. Smoking and lung function. Am Rev Respir Dis 1981;123(2):149–155.

22. Givelber RJ, Couropmitree NN, Gottlieb DJ, et al. Segregation analysis of pulmonary function among families in the Framingham Study. Am J Respir Crit Care Med 1998; 157(5 Pt 1):1445–1451.

23. Redline S, Tishler PV, Lewitter FI, Tager IB, Munoz a, Speizer FE. Assessment of genetic and nongenetic influences on pulmonary function. A twin study. Am Rev Respir Dis 1987;135(1):217–222.

24. Silverman EK. Genetics of chronic obstructive pulmonary disease. Novartis Found Symp 2001;234:45–58; discussion 58–64.

25. Sandford AJ, Pare PD. Genetic risk factors for chronic obstructive pulmonary disease. Clin Chest Med 2000;21(4):633–643.

26. Carrell RW, Jeppsson JO, Laurell CB, et al. Structure and variation of human alpha 1-antitrypsin. Nature 1982;298(5872):329–334.

27. Laurell CB, Eriksson S. The electrophoretic alpha1 globulin pattern of serum in alpha-1-antitrypsin deficiency. Scand J Clin Lab Invest 1963;15:133–140.

28. Eriksson S. A 30-year perspective on alpha 1-antitrypsin deficiency. Chest 1996;110(6 Suppl):237S–242S.

29. Lieberman J, Gaidulis L, Garoutte B, Mittman C. Identification and characteristics of the common alpha 1-antitrypsin phenotypes. Chest 1972;62(5):557–564.

30. Tobin MJ, Cook PJ, Hutchison DC. Alpha 1 antitrypsin deficiency: the clinical and physiological features of pulmonary emphysema in subjects homozygous for Pi type Z. A survey by the British Thoracic Association. Br J Dis Chest 1983;77(1):14–27.

31. Turino GM, Barker AF, Brantly ML, et al. Clinical features of individuals with PI*SZ phenotype of alpha 1-antitrypsin deficiency. Alpha 1-Antitrypsin Deficiency Registry Study Group. Am J Respir Crit Care Med 1996; 154(6 Pt 1):1718–1725.

32. Cox DW, Levison H. Emphysema of early onset associated with a complete deficiency of alpha-1-antitrypsin (null homozygotes). Am Rev Respir Dis 1988;137(2):371–375.

33. Seersholm N, Kok-Jensen A, Dirksen A. Survival of patients with severe alpha 1-antitrypsin deficiency with special reference to non-index cases. Thorax 1994;49(7):695–698.

34. Peto R, Speizer FE, Cochrane AL, et al. The relevance in adults of air-flow obstruction, but not of mucus hypersecretion, to mortality from chronic lung disease. Results from 20 years of prospective observation. Am Rev Respir Dis 1983;128(3):491–500.

35. Clement J, Van de Woestijne KP. Rapidly decreasing forced expiratory volume in one second or vital capacity and development of chronic airflow obstruction. Am Rev Respir Dis 1982;125(5):553–558.
36. Kanner RE, Renzetti AD, Jr, Klauber MR, Smith CB, Golden CA. Variables associated with changes in spirometry in patients with obstructive lung diseases. Am J Med 1979;67(1):44–50.
37. Lange P, Nyboe J, Appleyard M, Jensen G, Schnohr P. Relation of ventilatory impairment and of chronic mucus hypersecretion to mortality from obstructive lung disease and from all causes. Thorax 1990;45(8):579–585.
38. Kanner RE, Anthonisen NR, Connett JE. Lower respiratory illnesses promote FEV(1) decline in current smokers but not ex-smokers with mild chronic obstructive pulmonary disease. Results from the lung health study. Am J Respir Crit Care Med 2001;164(3):358–364.
39. Vestbo J, Prescott E, Lange P. Association of chronic mucus hypersecretion with FEV1 decline and chronic obstructive pulmonary disease morbidity. Copenhagen City Heart Study Group. Am J Respir Crit Care Med 1996;153(5):1530–1535.
40. Orie NG, Sluiter HJ, de Vries K, et al. The host factor in bronchitis. In: Orie NG, Sluiter HJ, eds. Bronchitis and International Symposium. Assen: Royal Vangorcum; 1961.
41. Tashkin DP, Altose MD, Connett JE, Kanner RE, Lee WW, Wise RA. Methacholine reactivity predicts changes in lung function over time in smokers with early chronic obstructive pulmonary disease. The Lung Health Study Research Group. Am J Respir Crit Care Med 1996; 153(6 Pt 1):1802–1811.
42. Cox BD. Blood pressure and respiratory function. In: The health and lifestyle survey. Preliminary report of a nationwide survey of the physical and mental health, attitudes and lifestyle of a random sample of 9003 British adults. London: Health Promotion Research Trust; 1987:17–33.
43. Seamark DA, Williams S, Timon S, et al. Home or surgery based screening for chronic obstructive pulmonary disease (COPD)? Prim Care Respir J 2001;10(2):30–33.
44. Office for National Statistics. Health Statistics Quarterly (8) Winter 2000. London: The Stationery Office; 2000.
45. Lopez AD, Murray CC. The global burden of disease, 1990–2020. Nat Med 1998;4(11):1241–1243.
46. Office of Population Census and Surveys. Morbidity Statistics from General Practice. Fourth national study 1991–1992. London: HMSO; 1995.
47. British Thoracic Society. The burden of lung disease. London: British Thoracic Society; 2001.
48. Mannino DM, Brown C, Giovino GA. Obstructive lung disease deaths in the United States from 1979 through 1993. An analysis using multiple-cause mortality data. Am J Respir Crit Care Med 1997;156(3 Pt 1):814–818.

Pathology and pathophysiology

49. Magee F, Wright JL, Wiggs BR, Pare PD, Hogg JC. Pulmonary vascular structure and function in chronic obstructive pulmonary disease. Thorax 1988;43(3):183–189.
50. Agusti AG. Systemic effects of chronic obstructive pulmonary disease. Novartis Found Symp 2001;234:242–249; discussion 250–254.
51. Saetta M, Turato G, Maestrelli P, Mapp CE, Fabbri LM. Cellular and structural bases of chronic obstructive pulmonary disease. Am J Respir Crit Care Med 2001;163(6):1304–1309.

52. Cosio MG, Hale KA, Niewoehner DE. Morphologic and morphometric effects of prolonged cigarette smoking on the small airways. Am Rev Respir Dis 1980;122(2):265–271.

53. Saetta M, Baraldo S, Corbino L, et al. CD8+ve cells in the lungs of smokers with chronic obstructive pulmonary disease. Am J Respir Crit Care Med 1999;160(2):711–717.

54. O'Shaughnessy TC, Ansari TW, Barnes NC, Jeffery PK. Inflammation in bronchial biopsies of subjects with chronic bronchitis: inverse relationship of CD8+ T lymphocytes with FEV1. Am J Respir Crit Care Med 1997;155(3):852–857.

55. MacNee W, Wiggs B, Belzberg AS, Hogg JC. The effect of cigarette smoking on neutrophil kinetics in human lungs. N Engl J Med 1989;321(14):924–928.

56. Saetta M, Di Stefano A, Maestrelli P, et al. Airway eosinophilia in chronic bronchitis during exacerbations. Am J Respir Crit Care Med 1994; 150(6 Pt 1):1646–1652.

57. Turato G, Di Stefano A, Maestrelli P, et al. Effect of smoking cessation on airway inflammation in chronic bronchitis. Am J Respir Crit Care Med 1995;152(4 Pt 1):1262–1267.

58. Rutgers SR, Postma DS, ten Hacken NH, et al. Ongoing airway inflammation in patients with COPD who do not currently smoke. Chest 2000;117(5 Suppl 1):262S.

59. Jeffery PK. Differences and similarities between chronic obstructive pulmonary disease and asthma. Clin Exp Allergy 1999;29(Suppl 2):14–26.

60. Medical Research Council. Definition and classification of chronic bronchitis for clinical and epidemiological purposes. A report to the Medical Research Council by their committee on the aetiology of chronic bronchitis. Lancet 1965;1:775–780.

61. Fletcher C, Peto R, Tinker C, Speizer F. The natural history of chronic bronchitis and emphysema. An 8 year study of working men. Oxford: Oxford University Press; 1976.

62. Peto R, Speizer FE, Cochrane AL, et al. The relevance in adults of air-flow obstruction, but not of mucus hypersecretion, to mortality from chronic lung disease. Results from 20 years of prospective observation. Am Rev Respir Dis 1983;128(3):491–500.

63. Snider GL, Kleinerman J, Thurlbeck WM. The definition of emphysema. Report of the National Heart, Lung and Blood Institute, Division of Lung Diseases Workshop. Am Rev Respir Dis 1985;132:182–185.

64. CIBA foundation guest symposium. Terminology, definitions and classification of chronic obstructive pulmonary emphysema and related conditions. Thorax 1959;14:286–299.

65. MacNee W. Pathophysiology of cor pulmonale in chronic obstructive pulmonary disease. Part One. Am J Respir Crit Care Med 1994;150(3):833–852.

66. Harris P, Heath D. The pulmonary vasculature in emphysema. In: Harris P, Heath D, eds. The human pulmonary circulation. Edinburgh: Churchill Livingstone; 1986:507–521.

67. Bignon J, Khoury F, Even P, Andre J, Brouet G. Morphometric study in chronic obstructive bronchopulmonary disease. Pathologic, clinical, and physiologic correlations. Am Rev Respir Dis 1969;99(5):669–695.

68. Hogg JC, Macklem PT, Thurlbeck WM. Site and nature of airway obstruction in chronic obstructive lung disease. N Engl J Med 1968;278(25):1355–1360.

69. Saetta M, Ghezzo H, Kim WD, et al. Loss of alveolar attachments in smokers. A morphometric correlate of

lung function impairment. Am Rev Respir Dis 1985;132(4):894–900.

70. Gibson GJ. Pulmonary hyperinflation: a clinical overview. Eur Respir J 1996;9(12):2640–2649.

71. Begin P, Grassino A. Inspiratory muscle dysfunction and chronic hypercapnia in chronic obstructive pulmonary disease. Am Rev Respir Dis 1991;143(5 Pt 1):905–912.

72. Agusti AG, Barbera JA. Contribution of multiple inert gas elimination technique to pulmonary medicine. 2. Chronic pulmonary diseases: chronic obstructive pulmonary disease and idiopathic pulmonary fibrosis. Thorax 1994;49(9):924–932.

73. Calverley P. Ventilatory control and dyspnea. In: Calverley P, Pride N, eds. Chronic obstructive pulmonary disease. London: Chapman & Hall; 1995:205–242.

74. Sassoon CS, Hassell KT, Mahutte CK. Hyperoxic-induced hypercapnia in stable chronic obstructive pulmonary disease. Am Rev Respir Dis 1987;135(4):907–911.

75. Aubier M, Murciano D, Milic-Emili J, et al. Effects of the administration of O2 on ventilation and blood gases in patients with chronic obstructive pulmonary disease during acute respiratory failure. Am Rev Respir Dis 1980;122(5):747–754.

76. Crossley DJ, McGuire GP, Barrow PM, Houston PL. Influence of inspired oxygen concentration on deadspace, respiratory drive, and PaCO2 in intubated patients with chronic obstructive pulmonary disease. Crit Care Med 1997;25(9):1522–1526.

77. Nunn JF, Milledge JS, Chen D, Dore C. Respiratory criteria of fitness for surgery and anaesthesia. Anaesthesia 1988;43(7):543–551.

78. Killian KJ, Leblanc P, Martin DH, Summers E, Jones NL, Campbell EJ.

Exercise capacity and ventilatory, circulatory, and symptom limitation in patients with chronic airflow limitation. Am Rev Respir Dis 1992;146(4):935–940.

79. O'Donnell DE, Revill SM, Webb KA. Dynamic hyperinflation and exercise intolerance in chronic obstructive pulmonary disease. Am J Respir Crit Care Med 2001;164(5):770–777.

80. Belman MJ. Exercise in patients with chronic obstructive pulmonary disease. Thorax 1993;48(9):936–946.

81. Tobin MJ. Respiratory muscles in disease. Clin Chest Med 1988;9(2):263–286.

82. Dantzker DR, D'Alonzo GE. The effect of exercise on pulmonary gas exchange in patients with severe chronic obstructive pulmonary disease. Am Rev Respir Dis 1986;134(6):1135–1139.

83. Gosselink R, Troosters T, Decramer M. Peripheral muscle weakness contributes to exercise limitation in COPD. Am J Respir Crit Care Med 1996;153(3):976–980.

84. Carter R, Nicotra B, Blevins W, Holiday D. Altered exercise gas exchange and cardiac function in patients with mild chronic obstructive pulmonary disease. Chest 1993;103(3):745–750.

85. Stubbing DG, Pengelly LD, Morse JL, Jones NL. Pulmonary mechanics during exercise in subjects with chronic airflow obstruction. J Appl Physiol 1980;49(3):511–515.

86. Bauerle O, Chrusch CA, Younes M. Mechanisms by which COPD affects exercise tolerance. Am J Respir Crit Care Med 1998;157(1):57–68.

87. Dodd DS, Brancatisano T, Engel LA. Chest wall mechanics during exercise in patients with severe chronic air-flow obstruction. Am Rev Respir Dis 1984;129(1):33–38.

88. Johnson BD, Reddan WG, Seow KC, Dempsey JA. Mechanical constraints on exercise hyperpnea in a fit aging population. Am Rev Respir Dis 1991;143(5 Pt 1):968–977.

89. Babb TG, Viggiano R, Hurley B, Staats B, Rodarte JR. Effect of mild-to-moderate airflow limitation on exercise capacity. J Appl Physiol 1991;70(1):223–230.

90. Skeletal muscle dysfunction in chronic obstructive pulmonary disease. A statement of the American Thoracic Society and European Respiratory Society. Am J Respir Crit Care Med 1999;159(4 Pt 2):S1–S40.

91. Engelen MP, Schols AM, Baken WC, Wesseling GJ, Wouters EF. Nutritional depletion in relation to respiratory and peripheral skeletal muscle function in out-patients with COPD. Eur Respir J 1994;7(10):1793–1797.

92. Steiner MC, Morgan MD. Enhancing physical performance in chronic obstructive pulmonary disease. Thorax 2001;56(1):73–77.

93. O'Donnell DE, Webb KA. Exertional breathlessness in patients with chronic airflow limitation. The role of lung hyperinflation. Am Rev Respir Dis 1993;148(5):1351–1357.

94. O'Donnell DE, Bertley JC, Chau LK, Webb KA. Qualitative aspects of exertional breathlessness in chronic airflow limitation: pathophysiologic mechanisms. Am J Respir Crit Care Med 1997;155(1):109–115.

95. Belman MJ, Botnick WC, Shin JW. Inhaled bronchodilators reduce dynamic hyperinflation during exercise in patients with chronic obstructive pulmonary disease. Am J Respir Crit Care Med 1996;153(3):967–975.

96. Martinez FJ, de Oca MM, Whyte RI, Stetz J, Gay SE, Celli BR. Lung-volume reduction improves dyspnea, dynamic hyperinflation, and respiratory muscle function. Am J Respir Crit Care Med 1997;155(6):1984–1990.

Diagnosis and prognosis

97. Zielinski J, Bednarek M. Early detection of COPD in a high-risk population using spirometric screening. Chest 2001;119(3):731–736.

98. Shigeoka JW. Calibration and quality control of spirometer systems. Respir Care 1983;28(6):747–753.

99. Nelson SB, Gardner RM, Crapo RO, Jensen RL. Performance evaluation of contemporary spirometers. Chest 1990;97(2):288–297.

100. Hankinson JL. State of the art of spirometric instrumentation. Chest 1990;97(2):258–259.

101. Ferguson GT, Enright PL, Buist AS, Higgins MW. Office spirometry for lung health assessment in adults: a consensus statement from the national lung health education program. Chest 2000;117(4):1146–1161.

102. Tablan OC, Williams WW, Martone WJ. Infection control in pulmonary function laboratories. Infect Control 1985;6(11):442–444.

103. Standardization of Spirometry, 1994 Update. American Thoracic Society. Am J Respir Crit Care Med 1995;152(3):1107–1136.

104. Guidelines for the measurement of respiratory function. Recommendations of the British Thoracic Society and the Association of Respiratory Technicians and Physiologists. Respir Med 1994;88(3):165–194.

105. Quanjer PH, Tammeling GJ, Cotes JE, Pedersen OF, Peslin R, Yernault JC. Lung volumes and forced ventilatory flows. Report of the Working Party on Standardization of Lung Function Tests, European Community for Steel and Coal. Official Statement of the

European Respiratory Society. Eur Respir J Suppl 1993;16:5–40.

106. Tweeddale PM, Alexander F, McHardy GJ. Short term variability in FEV1 and bronchodilator responsiveness in patients with obstructive ventilatory defects. Thorax 1987;42(7):487–490.

107. Nolan D, White P, Pearson MG. FEV-1 and PEF in COPD management. Thorax 1999;54(5):468–469.

108. Brand PL, Quanjer PH, Postma DS, et al. Interpretation of bronchodilator response in patients with obstructive airways disease. The Dutch Chronic Non Specific Lung Disease (CNSLD) Study Group. Thorax 1992;47(6):429–436.

109. MacNee W. Consensus conference on management of chronic obstructive pulmonary disease. J R Coll Physicians Edinb 2002;32(Suppl 10):1–46.

110. Hay JG, Stone P, Carter J, et al. Bronchodilator reversibility, exercise performance and breathlessness in stable chronic obstructive pulmonary disease. Eur Respir J 1992;5(6):659–664.

111. Kerstjens HA, Brand PL, Quanjer PH, van der Bruggen-Bogaarts BA, Koeter GH, Postma DS. Variability of bronchodilator response and effects of inhaled corticosteroid treatment in obstructive airways disease. Dutch CNSLD Study Group. Thorax 1993;48(7):722–729.

112. Burge PS, Calverley PM, Jones PW, Spencer S, Anderson JA, Maslen TK. Randomised, double blind, placebo controlled study of fluticasone propionate in patients with moderate to severe chronic obstructive pulmonary disease: the ISOLDE trial. BMJ 2000;320(7245):1297–1303.

113. Cazzola M, Vinciguerra A, Di Perna F, Matera MG. Early reversibility to salbutamol does not always predict bronchodilation after salmeterol in stable chronic obstructive pulmonary disease. Respir Med 1998;92(8):1012–1016.

114. Rimmington LD, Nisar M, Earis JE, Calverley PMA, Pearson MG. Predictors of 5 year mortality in COPD. Am Rev Respir Dis 1993;147:A323.

115. Calverley PM. Symptomatic bronchodilator treatment. In: Calverley PM, Pride N, eds. Chronic obstructive pulmonary disease. London: Chapman & Hall; 1995:419–445.

116. Pauwels RA, Buist AS, Calverley PM, Jenkins CR, Hurd SS. Global strategy for the diagnosis, management, and prevention of chronic obstructive pulmonary disease. NHLBI/WHO Global Initiative for Chronic Obstructive Lung Disease (GOLD) Workshop summary. Am J Respir Crit Care Med 2001;163(5):1256–1276.

117. Standards for the diagnosis and care of patients with chronic obstructive pulmonary disease. American Thoracic Society. Am J Respir Crit Care Med 1995;152(5 Pt 2):S77–S121.

118. Siafakas NM, Vermeire P, Pride NB, et al. Optimal assessment and management of chronic obstructive pulmonary disease (COPD). The European Respiratory Society Task Force. Eur Respir J 1995;8(8):1398–1420.

119. Schermer TRJ, Folgering HTM, Bottema B, Jacobs JE, Van Schayck CP, Van Weel C. The value of spirometry for primary care: Asthma and COPD. Asthma Gen Pract 2000;9(3):51–55.

120. Weisman IM, Zeballos RJ. Clinical exercise testing. Clin Chest Med 2001;22(4):679–701, viii.

121. Butland RJ, Pang J, Gross ER, Woodcock AA, Geddes DM. Two-, six-, and 12-minute walking tests in respiratory disease. BMJ (Clin Res Ed) 1982;284(6329):1607–1608.

122. ATS statement: guidelines for the six-minute walk test. Am J Respir Crit Care Med 2002;166(1):111–117.

123. Redelmeier DA, Bayoumi AM, Goldstein RS, Guyatt GH. Interpreting small differences in functional status: the six minute walk test in chronic lung disease patients. Am J Respir Crit Care Med 1997;155(4):1278–1282.

124. Guyatt GH, Pugsley SO, Sullivan MJ, et al. Effect of encouragement on walking test performance. Thorax 1984;39(11):818–822.

125. Singh SJ, Morgan MD, Scott S, Walters D, Hardman AE. Development of a shuttle walking test of disability in patients with chronic airways obstruction. Thorax 1992;47(12):1019–1024.

126. Revill SM, Morgan MD, Singh SJ, Williams J, Hardman AE. The endurance shuttle walk: a new field test for the assessment of endurance capacity in chronic obstructive pulmonary disease. Thorax 1999;54(3):213–222.

127. Fletcher C, Peto R, Tinker C, Speizer F. The natural history of chronic bronchitis and emphysema. An 8 year study of working men. Oxford: Oxford University Press; 1976.

128. Burrows B, Earle RH. Course and prognosis of chronic obstructive lung disease. A prospective study of 200 patients. N Engl J Med 1969;280(8):397–404.

129. Scanlon PD, Connett JE, Waller LA, Altose MD, Bailey WC, Buist AS. Smoking cessation and lung function in mild-to-moderate chronic obstructive pulmonary disease. The Lung Health Study. Am J Respir Crit Care Med 2000;161(2 Pt 1):381–390.

130. Mannino DM, Gagnon RC, Petty TL, Lydick E. Obstructive lung disease and low lung function in adults in the United States: data from the National Health and Nutrition Examination Survey, 1988–1994. Arch Intern Med 2000;160(11):1683–1689.

131. Vestbo J, Lange P. Can GOLD Stage 0 provide information of prognostic value in chronic obstructive pulmonary disease? Am J Respir Crit Care Med 2002;166(3):329–332.

132. Soriano JB, Maier WC, Egger P, et al. Recent trends in physician diagnosed COPD in women and men in the UK. Thorax 2000;55(9):789–794.

133. Burrows B, Earle RH. Chronic obstructive lung disease. N Engl J Med 1969;280(21):1183–1184.

134. Keistinen T, Tuuponen T, Kivela SL. Survival experience of the population needing hospital treatment for asthma or COPD at age 50–54 years. Respir Med 1998;92(3):568–572.

135. Vilkman S, Keistinen T, Tuuponen T, Kivela SL. Survival and cause of death among elderly chronic obstructive pulmonary disease patients after first admission to hospital. Respiration 1997;64(4):281–284.

136. Nishimura K, Tsukino M. Clinical course and prognosis of patients with chronic obstructive pulmonary disease. Curr Opin Pulm Med 2000;6(2):127–132.

137. Traver GA, Cline MG, Burrows B. Predictors of mortality in chronic obstructive pulmonary disease. A 15-year follow-up study. Am Rev Respir Dis 1979;119(6):895–902.

138. Thomason MJ, Strachan DP. Which spirometric indices best predict subsequent death from chronic obstructive pulmonary disease? Thorax 2000;55(9):785–788.

139. Schols AM, Soeters PB, Dingemans AM, Mostert R, Frantzen PJ, Wouters EF. Prevalence and characteristics of nutritional depletion in patients with stable COPD eligible for pulmonary rehabilitation. Am Rev Respir Dis 1993;147(5):1151–1156.

140. Gray-Donald K, Gibbons L, Shapiro SH, Macklem PT, Martin JG.

Nutritional status and mortality in chronic obstructive pulmonary disease. Am J Respir Crit Care Med 1996;153(3):961–966.

141. Marquis K, Debigare R, Lacasse Y, et al. Midthigh muscle cross-sectional area is a better predictor of mortality than body mass index in patients with chronic obstructive pulmonary disease. Am J Respir Crit Care Med 2002;166:809–913.

142. Fletcher CM, Elmes PC, Wood CI. The significance of respiratory symptoms and the diagnosis of chronic bronchitis in a working population. BMJ 1959;2:257–266.

143. Nishimura K, Izumi T, Tsukino M, Oga T. Dyspnea is a better predictor of 5-year survival than airway obstruction in patients with COPD. Chest 2002;121(5):1434–1440.

144. Anthonisen NR, Wright EC, Hodgkin JE. Prognosis in chronic obstructive pulmonary disease. Am Rev Respir Dis 1986;133(1):14–20.

145. Domingo-Salvany A, Lamarca R, Ferrer M, et al. Health-related quality of life and mortality in male patients with chronic obstructive pulmonary disease. Am J Respir Crit Care Med 2002;166(5):680–685.

146. Burrows B, Earle RH. Predictors of survival in patients with chronic airways obstruction. Am Rev Respir Dis 1969;99:865–871.

147. Boushy SF, Thompson HK, Jr, North LB, Beale AR, Snow TR. Prognosis in chronic obstructive pulmonary disease. Am Rev Respir Dis 1973;108(6):1373–1383.

148. Dubois P, Machiels J, Smeets F, Delwiche JP, Lulling J. CO transfer capacity as a determining factor of survival for severe hypoxaemic COPD patients under long-term oxygen therapy. Eur Respir J 1990;3(9):1042–1047.

149. Chailleux E, Fauroux B, Binet F, Dautzenberg B, Polu JM. Predictors of survival in patients receiving domiciliary oxygen therapy or mechanical ventilation. A 10-year analysis of ANTADIR Observatory. Chest 1996;109(3):741–749.

150. Vandenbergh E, Clement J, Van de Woestijne KP. Course and prognosis of patients with advanced chronic obstructive pulmonary disease. Evaluation by means of functional indices. Am J Med 1973;55(6):736–746.

151. Klinger JR, Hill NS. Right ventricular dysfunction in chronic obstructive pulmonary disease. Evaluation and management. Chest 1991; 99(3):715–723.

Management guidelines for COPD

152. COPD Guidelines Group of the Standards of Care Committee of the BTS. BTS guidelines for the management of chronic obstructive pulmonary disease. Thorax 1997;52(Suppl 5):S1–28.

153. American Thoracic Society. Standards for the diagnosis and care of patients with chronic obstructive pulmonary disease. Am J Respir Crit Care Med 1995;152(5 Pt 2):S77–S121.

154. Siafakas NM, Vermeire P, Pride NB, et al. Optimal assessment and management of chronic obstructive pulmonary disease (COPD). The European Respiratory Society Task Force. Eur Respir J 1995;8(8):1398–1420.

155. Pauwels RA, Buist AS, Calverley PM, Jenkins CR, Hurd SS. Global strategy for the diagnosis, management, and prevention of chronic obstructive pulmonary disease. NHLBI/WHO Global Initiative for Chronic Obstructive Lung Disease (GOLD) Workshop summary. Am J Respir Crit Care Med 2001;163(5):1256–1276.

156. O'Donnell DE. Assessment of bronchodilator efficacy in symptomatic COPD: is spirometry useful? Chest 2000; 117(2 Suppl):42S–47S.

157. Spencer S, Calverley PM, Sherwood Burge P, Jones PW. Health status deterioration in patients with chronic obstructive pulmonary disease. Am J Respir Crit Care Med 2001;163(1):122–128.

Prevention of COPD

158. Fletcher C, Peto R, Tinker C, Speizer F. The natural history of chronic bronchitis and emphysema. An 8 year study of working men. Oxford: Oxford University Press; 1976.

159. Scanlon PD, Connett JE, Waller LA, Altose MD, Bailey WC, Buist AS. Smoking cessation and lung function in mild-to-moderate chronic obstructive pulmonary disease. The Lung Health Study. Am J Respir Crit Care Med 2000; 161(2 Pt 1):381–390.

160. Warner KE. Cost effectiveness of smoking-cessation therapies. Interpretation of the evidence and implications for coverage. Pharmacoeconomics 1997; 11(6):538–549.

161. Cohen D, Barton G. The cost to society of smoking cessation. Thorax 1998;53(Suppl 2):S38–S42.

162. West R, McNeill A, Raw M. Smoking cessation guidelines for health professionals: an update. Health Education Authority. Thorax 2000;55(12):987–999.

163. Lillington GA, Leonard CT, Sachs DP. Smoking cessation. Techniques and benefits. Clin Chest Med 2000;21(1):199–208, xi.

164. Tashkin D, Kanner R, Bailey W, et al. Smoking cessation in patients with chronic obstructive pulmonary disease: a double-blind, placebo-controlled, randomised trial. Lancet 2001;357(9268):1571–1575.

165. Hepper NG, Drage CW, Davies SF, et al. Chronic obstructive pulmonary disease: a community-oriented program including professional education and screening by a voluntary health agency. Am Rev Respir Dis 1980;121(1):97–104.

166. Risser NL, Belcher DW. Adding spirometry, carbon monoxide, and pulmonary symptom results to smoking cessation counseling: a randomized trial. J Gen Intern Med 1990;5(1):16–22.

167. Humerfelt S, Eide GE, Kvale G, Aaro LE, Gulsvik A. Effectiveness of postal smoking cessation advice: a randomized controlled trial in young men with reduced FEV1 and asbestos exposure. Eur Respir J 1998;11(2):284–290.

168. Czajkowska-Malinowska M, Bednarek M, Zielinski J. Effects of repeated spirometry combined with an antismoking advice on smoking cessation rate. Am J Respir Crit Care Med 2001;163(5):A355.

169. Wilcke JT. Late onset genetic disease: where ignorance is bliss, is it folly to inform relatives? BMJ 1998;317(7160):744–747.

Drug therapy

170. COPD Guidelines Group of the Standards of Care Committee of the BTS. BTS guidelines for the management of chronic obstructive pulmonary disease. Thorax 1997;52(Suppl 5):S1–28.

171. Pauwels RA, Buist AS, Calverley PM, Jenkins CR, Hurd SS. Global strategy for the diagnosis, management, and prevention of chronic obstructive pulmonary disease. NHLBI/WHO Global Initiative for Chronic Obstructive Lung Disease (GOLD)

Workshop summary. Am J Respir Crit Care Med 2001;163(5):1256–1276.

172. Corris PA, Neville E, Nariman S, Gibson GJ. Dose–response study of inhaled salbutamol powder in chronic airflow obstruction. Thorax 1983;38(4):292–296.

173. Teale C, Morrison JF, Page RL, Pearson SB. Dose response to inhaled salbutamol in chronic obstructive airways disease. Postgrad Med J 1991;67(790):754–756.

174. Sestini P, Renzoni E, Robinson S, Poole P, Ram FS. Short-acting beta 2 agonists for stable COPD (Cochrane review). Cochrane Database Syst Rev 2000;(3):CD001495.

175. Nelson HS. Beta-adrenergic bronchodilators. N Engl J Med 1995;333(8):499–506.

176. Bengtsson B. Plasma concentration and side-effects of terbutaline. Eur J Respir Dis Suppl 1984;134:231–235.

177. Teule GJ, Majid PA. Haemodynamic effects of terbutaline in chronic obstructive airways disease. Thorax 1980;35(7):536–542.

178. Harris L. Comparison of the effect on blood gases, ventilation, and perfusion of isoproterenol-phenylephrine and salbutamol aerosols in chronic bronchitis with asthma. J Allergy Clin Immunol 1972;49(2):63–71.

179. Weber RW, Smith JA, Nelson HS. Aerosolized terbutaline in asthmatics: development of subsensitivity with long-term administration. J Allergy Clin Immunol 1982;70(6):417–422.

180. Repsher LH, Anderson JA, Bush RK, et al. Assessment of tachyphylaxis following prolonged therapy of asthma with inhaled albuterol aerosol. Chest 1984;85(1):34–38.

181. Nicklas RA. Paradoxical bronchospasm associated with the use of inhaled beta agonists. J Allergy Clin Immunol 1990;85(5):959–964.

182. Gross NJ, Co E, Skorodin MS. Cholinergic bronchomotor tone in COPD. Estimates of its amount in comparison with that in normal subjects. Chest 1989;96(5):984–987.

183. Minette PA, Barnes PJ. Muscarinic receptor subtypes in lung. Clinical implications. Am Rev Respir Dis 1990;141(3 Pt 2):S162–S165.

184. Burge PS, Harries MG, l'Anson E. Comparison of atropine with ipratropium bromide in patients with reversible airways obstruction unresponsive to salbutamol. Br J Dis Chest 1980;74(3):259–262.

185. Easton PA, Jadue C, Dhingra S, Anthonisen NR. A comparison of the bronchodilating effects of a beta-2 adrenergic agent (albuterol) and an anticholinergic agent (ipratropium bromide), given by aerosol alone or in sequence. N Engl J Med 1986;315(12):735–739.

186. Braun SR, Levy SF. Comparison of ipratropium bromide and albuterol in chronic obstructive pulmonary disease: a three-center study. Am J Med 1991;91(4A):28S–32S.

187. COMBIVENT Inhalation Aerosol Study Group. In chronic obstructive pulmonary disease, a combination of ipratropium and albuterol is more effective than either agent alone. An 85-day multicenter trial. Chest 1994;105(5):1411–1419.

188. Martin RJ, Bartelson BL, Smith P, et al. Effect of ipratropium bromide treatment on oxygen saturation and sleep quality in COPD. Chest 1999;115(5):1338–1345.

189. Gross NJ. Ipratropium bromide. N Engl J Med 1988;319(8):486–494.

190. Anderson WM. Hemodynamic and non bronchial effects of ipratropium bromide. Am J Med 1986;81(5A):45–53.

191. Connolly CK. Adverse reaction to ipratropium bromide. BMJ (Clin Res Ed) 1982;285(6346):934–935.

192. Johnson M, Rennard S. Alternative mechanisms for long-acting beta(2)-adrenergic agonists in COPD. Chest 2001;120(1):258–270.

193. Appleton S, Smith B, Veale A, Bara A. Long-acting beta2-agonists for chronic obstructive pulmonary disease. Cochrane Database Syst Rev 2000;(2):CD001104.

194. Rennard SI, Anderson W, ZuWallack R, et al. Use of a long-acting inhaled beta2-adrenergic agonist, salmeterol xinafoate, in patients with chronic obstructive pulmonary disease. Am J Respir Crit Care Med 2001;163(5):1087–1092.

195. van Noord JA, de Munck DR, Bantje TA, Hop WC, Akveld ML, Bommer AM. Long-term treatment of chronic obstructive pulmonary disease with salmeterol and the additive effect of ipratropium. Eur Respir J 2000;15(5):878–885.

196. Jones PW, Bosh TK. Quality of life changes in COPD patients treated with salmeterol. Am J Respir Crit Care Med 1997;155(4):1283–1289.

197. Dahl R, Greefhorst LA, Nowak D, et al. Inhaled formoterol dry powder versus ipratropium bromide in chronic obstructive pulmonary disease. Am J Respir Crit Care Med 2001;164(5):778–784.

198. Cazzola M, Imperatore F, Salzillo A, et al. Cardiac effects of formoterol and salmeterol in patients suffering from COPD with preexisting cardiac arrhythmias and hypoxemia. Chest 1998;114(2):411–415.

199. Cheung D, Timmers MC, Zwinderman AH, Bel EH, Dijkman JH, Sterk PJ. Long-term effects of a long-acting beta 2-adrenoceptor agonist, salmeterol, on airway hyperresponsiveness in patients with mild asthma. N Engl J Med 1992;327(17):1198–1203.

200. Donohue JF, van Noord JA, Bateman ED, et al. A 6-month, placebo-controlled study comparing lung function and health status changes in COPD patients treated with tiotropium or salmeterol. Chest 2002;122(1):47–55.

201. Littner MR, Ilowite JS, Tashkin DP, et al. Long-acting bronchodilation with once-daily dosing of tiotropium (Spiriva) in stable chronic obstructive pulmonary disease. Am J Respir Crit Care Med 2000;161(4 Pt 1):1136–1142.

202. Barnes PJ. The pharmacological properties of tiotropium. Chest 2000;117(2 Suppl):63S–66S.

203. Casaburi R, Briggs DD, Jr, Donohue JF, Serby CW, Menjoge SS, Witek TJ, Jr. The spirometric efficacy of once-daily dosing with tiotropium in stable COPD: a 13-week multicenter trial. Chest 2000;118(5):1294–1302.

204. van Noord JA, Bantje TA, Eland ME, Korducki L, Cornelissen PJ. A randomised controlled comparison of tiotropium and ipratropium in the treatment of chronic obstructive pulmonary disease. The Dutch Tiotropium Study Group. Thorax 2000;55(4):289–294.

205. Keatings VM, Jatakanon A, Worsdell YM, Barnes PJ. Effects of inhaled and oral glucocorticoids on inflammatory indices in asthma and COPD. Am J Respir Crit Care Med 1997;155(2):542–548.

206. Hattotuwa KL, Gizycki MJ, Ansari TW, Jeffery PK, Barnes NC. The effects of inhaled fluticasone on airway inflammation in chronic obstructive pulmonary disease: a double-blind, placebo-controlled biopsy study. Am J Respir Crit Care Med 2002;165(12):1592–1596.

207. Burge PS, Calverley PM, Jones PW, Spencer S, Anderson JA, Maslen TK. Randomised, double blind, placebo controlled study of fluticasone propionate in patients with moderate

to severe chronic obstructive pulmonary disease: the ISOLDE trial. BMJ 2000;320(7245):1297–1303.

208. The Lung Health Study Research Group. Effect of inhaled triamcinolone on the decline in pulmonary function in chronic obstructive pulmonary disease. N Engl J Med 2000;343(26):1902–1909.

209. Vestbo J, Sorensen T, Lange P, Brix A, Torre P, Viskum K. Long-term effect of inhaled budesonide in mild and moderate chronic obstructive pulmonary disease: a randomised controlled trial. Lancet 1999;353(9167):1819–1823.

210. Pauwels RA, Lofdahl CG, Laitinen LA, et al. Long-term treatment with inhaled budesonide in persons with mild chronic obstructive pulmonary disease who continue smoking. European Respiratory Society Study on Chronic Obstructive Pulmonary Disease. N Engl J Med 1999;340(25):1948–1953.

211. Paggiaro PL, Dahle R, Bakran I, Frith L, Hollingworth K, Efthimiou J. Multicentre randomised placebo-controlled trial of inhaled fluticasone propionate in patients with chronic obstructive pulmonary disease. International COPD Study Group. Lancet 1998;351(9105):773–780.

212. McEvoy CE, Niewoehner DE. Adverse effects of corticosteroid therapy for COPD. A critical review. Chest 1997;111(3):732–743.

213. Chanez P, Vignola AM, O'Shaugnessy T, et al. Corticosteroid reversibility in COPD is related to features of asthma. Am J Respir Crit Care Med 1997;155(5):1529–1534.

214. Senderovitz T, Vestbo J, Frandsen J, et al. Steroid reversibility test followed by inhaled budesonide or placebo in outpatients with stable chronic obstructive pulmonary disease. The Danish Society of Respiratory

Medicine. Respir Med 1999; 93(10):715–718.

215. Callahan CM, Dittus RS, Katz BP. Oral corticosteroid therapy for patients with stable chronic obstructive pulmonary disease. A meta-analysis. Ann Intern Med 1991;114(3):216–223.

216. Weir DC, Gove RI, Robertson AS, Burge PS. Corticosteroid trials in non-asthmatic chronic airflow obstruction: a comparison of oral prednisolone and inhaled beclomethasone dipropionate. Thorax 1990;45(2):112–117.

217. Lightbody IM, Ingram CG, Legge JS, Johnston RN. Ipratropium bromide, salbutamol and prednisolone in bronchial asthma and chronic bronchitis. Br J Dis Chest 1978;72(3):181–186.

218. Douglas NJ, Davidson I, Sudlow MF, Flenley DC. Bronchodilatation and the site of airway resistance in severe chronic bronchitis. Thorax 1979;34(1):51–56.

219. Ikeda A, Nishimura K, Koyama H, Izumi T. Bronchodilating effects of combined therapy with clinical dosages of ipratropium bromide and salbutamol for stable COPD: comparison with ipratropium bromide alone. Chest 1995;107(2):401–405.

220. Wesseling G, Mostert R, Wouters EF. A comparison of the effects of anticholinergic and beta 2-agonist and combination therapy on respiratory impedance in COPD. Chest 1992;101(1):166–173.

221. Chan CS, Brown IG, Kelly CA, Dent AG, Zimmerman PV. Bronchodilator responses to nebulised ipratropium and salbutamol singly and in combination in chronic bronchitis. Br J Clin Pharmacol 1984;17(1):103–105.

222. Higgins BG, Powell RM, Cooper S, Tattersfield AE. Effect of salbutamol and ipratropium bromide on airway calibre and bronchial reactivity in

asthma and chronic bronchitis. Eur Respir J 1991;4(4):415–420.

223. Mahler DA, Wong E, Giessel G, et al. Improvements in FEV1 and symptoms in COPD patients following 24 weeks of twice daily treatment with salmeterol 50/fluticasone proprionate 500 combination. Am J Respir Crit Care Med 2001;163(5):A279.

224. Hanania NA, Ramsdell J, Payne K, et al. Improvements in airflow and dyspnea in COPD patients following 24 weeks treatment with salmeterol 50mg and fluticasone proprionate 250mg alone or in combination via the diskus. Am J Respir Crit Care Med 2001;163(5):A279.

225. Calverley P, Pauwels R, Vestbo J. Salmeterol/fluticasone propionate combination for one year provides greater clinical benefit than its individual components in COPD. Am J Respir Crit Care Med 2002;165(8):A226.

226. Pauwels R, Calverley P, Vestbo J, et al. Reduction of exacerbations with salmeterol/fluticasone combination 50/500 mcg bd in the treatment of COPD. Eur Respir J 2002;20(Suppl 38):241S.

227. Dahl R, Cukier A, Olsson H. Budesonide/formoterol in a single inhaler reduces severe and mild exacerbations in patients with moderate to severe COPD. Eur Respir J 2002;20(Suppl 38):242S.

228. Jones P, Stahl E, Svensson K. Improvement in health status in patients with moderate to severe COPD after treatment with budesonide/formerol in a single inhaler. Eur Respir J 2002;20(Suppl 38):250S.

229. Mahler DA, Wire P, Horstman D, et al. Effectiveness of fluticasone propionate and salmeterol combination delivered via the diskus device in the treatment of chronic obstructive pulmonary disease. Am J Respir Crit Care Med 2002;166(8):1084–1091.

230. Calverley P, Pauwels R, Vestbo J, et al. Combined salmeterol and fluticasone in the treatment of chronic obstructive pulmonary disease: a randomised controlled trial. Lancet 2003;361(9356):449–456.

231. Vaz Fragoso CA, Miller MA. Review of the clinical efficacy of theophylline in the treatment of chronic obstructive pulmonary disease. Am Rev Respir Dis 1993;147(6 Pt 2):S40–S47.

232. Vassallo R, Lipsky JJ. Theophylline: recent advances in the understanding of its mode of action and uses in clinical practice. Mayo Clin Proc 1998;73(4):346–354.

233. Ramsdell J. Use of theophylline in the treatment of COPD. Chest 1995; 107(5 Suppl):206S–209S.

234. Murciano D, Aubier M, Lecocguic Y, Pariente R. Effects of theophylline on diaphragmatic strength and fatigue in patients with chronic obstructive pulmonary disease. N Engl J Med 1984;311(6):349–353.

235. Ziment I. Theophylline and mucociliary clearance. Chest 1987; 92(1 Suppl):38S–43S.

236. Matthay RA, Mahler DA. Theophylline improves global cardiac function and reduces dyspnea in chronic obstructive lung disease. J Allergy Clin Immunol 1986;78(4 Pt 2):793–799.

237. Lakshminarayan S, Sahn SA, Weil JV. Effect of aminophylline on ventilatory responses in normal man. Am Rev Respir Dis 1978;117(1):33–38.

238. Sanders JS, Berman TM, Bartlett MM, Kronenberg RS. Increased hypoxic ventilatory drive due to administration of aminophylline in normal men. Chest 1980;78(2):279–282.

239. Sharp JT. Theophylline in chronic obstructive pulmonary disease. J Allergy Clin Immunol 1986;78(4 Pt 2):800–805.

240. Chrystyn H, Mulley BA, Peake MD. Dose response relation to oral theophylline in severe chronic obstructive airways disease. BMJ 1988;297(6662):1506–1510.

241. Murciano D, Auclair MH, Pariente R, Aubier M. A randomized, controlled trial of theophylline in patients with severe chronic obstructive pulmonary disease. N Engl J Med 1989;320(23):1521–1525.

242. Tsukino M, Nishimura K, Ikeda A, Hajiro T, Koyama H, Izumi T. Effects of theophylline and ipratropium bromide on exercise performance in patients with stable chronic obstructive pulmonary disease. Thorax 1998;53(4):269–273.

243. Cazzola M, Donner CF, Matera MG. Long acting beta(2) agonists and theophylline in stable chronic obstructive pulmonary disease. Thorax 1999;54(8):730–736.

244. Karpel JP, Kotch A, Zinny M, Pesin J, Alleyne W. A comparison of inhaled ipratropium, oral theophylline plus inhaled beta-agonist, and the combination of all three in patients with COPD. Chest 1994;105(4):1089–1094.

245. Upton RA. Pharmacokinetic interactions between theophylline and other medication (Part I). Clin Pharmacokinet 1991;20(1):66–80.

246. Aronson JK, Hardman M, Reynolds DJ. ABC of monitoring drug therapy. Theophylline. BMJ 1992; 305(6865):1355–1358.

247. Halpin DMG, Hart E, Harris T, Harbour R, Rudolf M. What do general practice records tell us about the current management of COPD and the impact of the BTS COPD guidelines? Thorax 2000;55(Suppl 3):A38.

248. Ram FSF, Jones P, Castro AA, et al. Oral theophylline for chronic obstructive pulmonary disease (Cochrane Review). Cochrane Database Syst Rev 2002;(4):CD003902.

249. Guyatt GH, Townsend M, Pugsley SO, et al. Bronchodilators in chronic air-flow limitation. Effects on airway function, exercise capacity, and quality of life. Am Rev Respir Dis 1987;135(5):1069–1074.

250. Shannon M, Lovejoy FH, Jr. The influence of age vs peak serum concentration on life-threatening events after chronic theophylline intoxication. Arch Intern Med 1990;150(10):2045–2048.

251. Connolly MJ. Inhaler technique of elderly patients: comparison of metered-dose inhalers and large volume spacer devices. Age Ageing 1995;24(3):190–192.

252. Allen SC, Prior A. What determines whether an elderly patient can use a metered dose inhaler correctly? Br J Dis Chest 1986;80(1):45–49.

253. Mestitz H, Copland JM, App B, McDonald CF. Comparison of outpatient nebulised vs metered dose inhaler terbutaline in chronic airflow obstruction. Chest 1989;96:1237–1240.

254. Gross NJ, Petty TL, Friedman M, Skorodin MS, Silvers GW, Donohue JF. Dose response to ipratropium as a nebulized solution in patients with chronic obstructive pulmonary disease. A three-center study. Am Rev Respir Dis 1989;139(5):1188–1191.

255. O'Driscoll BR, Kay EA, Taylor RJ, Weatherby H, Chetty MC, Bernstein A. A long-term prospective assessment of home nebulizer treatment. Respir Med 1992;86(4):317–325.

256. Wilson RSE, Connellan SJ. Domiciliary nebulised salbutamol solution in severe chronic airway obstruction. Thorax 1980;35:873–876.

257. Morrison JF, Jones PC, Muers MF. Assessing physiological benefit from domiciliary nebulized bronchodilators

in severe airflow limitation. Eur Respir J 1992;5(4):424–429.

258. Gunawardena KA, Smith AP, Shankleman J. A comparison of metered dose inhalers with nebulizers from the delivery of ipratropium bromide in domiciliary practice. Br J Dis Chest 1986;80(2):170–178.

259. Jenkins SC, Heaton RW, Fulton TJ, Moxham J. Comparison of domiciliary nebulized salbutamol and salbutamol from a metered-dose inhaler in stable chronic airflow limitation. Chest 1987;91(6):804–807.

260. O'Driscoll BR. Nebulisers for chronic obstructive pulmonary disease. Thorax 1997;52(Suppl 2):S49–S52.

261. ZuWallack RL, Mahler DA, Reilly D, et al. Salmeterol plus theophylline combination therapy in the treatment of COPD. Chest 2001;119(6):1661–1670.

Treating exacerbations of COPD

262. Seemungal TA, Donaldson GC, Paul EA, Bestall JC, Jeffries DJ, Wedzicha JA. Effect of exacerbation on quality of life in patients with chronic obstructive pulmonary disease. Am J Respir Crit Care Med 1998;157(5 Pt 1):1418–1422.

263. Donaldson GC, Seemungal T, Jeffries DJ, Wedzicha JA. Effect of temperature on lung function and symptoms in chronic obstructive pulmonary disease. Eur Respir J 1999;13(4):844–849.

264. Wedzicha JA. Mechanisms of exacerbations. Novartis Found Symp 2001;234:84–93; discussion 93–103.

265. Wilson R. Bacteria, antibiotics and COPD. Eur Respir J 2001;17(5):995–1007.

266. Murphy TF, Sethi S, Niederman MS. The role of bacteria in exacerbations of COPD. A constructive view. Chest 2000;118(1):204–209.

267. Garcia-Aymerich J, Monso E, Marrades RM, et al. Risk factors for hospitalization for a chronic obstructive pulmonary disease exacerbation. EFRAM study. Am J Respir Crit Care Med 2001;164(6):1002–1007.

268. Burge PS, Calverley PM, Jones PW, Spencer S, Anderson JA, Maslen TK. Randomised, double blind, placebo controlled study of fluticasone propionate in patients with moderate to severe chronic obstructive pulmonary disease: the ISOLDE trial. BMJ 2000;320(7245):1297–1303.

269. Calverley P, Pauwels R, Vestbo J, et al. Combined salmeterol and fluticasone in the treatment of chronic obstructive pulmonary disease: a randomised controlled trial. Lancet 2003;361(9356):449–456.

270. Vincken W, van Noord JA, Greefhorst AP, et al. Improved health outcomes in patients with COPD during 1 yr's treatment with tiotropium. Eur Respir J 2002;19(2):209–216.

271. Casaburi R, Mahler DA, Jones PW, et al. A long-term evaluation of once-daily inhaled tiotropium in chronic obstructive pulmonary disease. Eur Respir J 2002;19(2):217–224.

272. Killen J, Ellis H. Assisted discharge for patients with exacerbations of chronic obstructive pulmonary disease: safe and effective. Thorax 2000;55(11):885.

273. Gravil JH, Al-Rawas OA, Cotton MM, Flanigan U, Irwin A, Stevenson RD. Home treatment of exacerbations of chronic obstructive pulmonary disease by an acute respiratory assessment service. Lancet 1998;351(9119):1853–1855.

274. Shepperd S, Harwood D, Jenkinson C, Gray A, Vessey M, Morgan P. Randomised controlled trial comparing hospital at home care with inpatient hospital care. I: three month follow up of health outcomes BMJ 1998;316(7147):1786–1791.

275. Shepperd S, Harwood D, Gray A, Vessey M, Morgan P. Randomised

controlled trial comparing hospital at home care with inpatient hospital care. II: cost minimisation analysis. BMJ 1998;316(7147):1791–1796.

276. Cotton MM, Bucknall CE, Dagg KD, et al. Early discharge for patients with exacerbations of chronic obstructive pulmonary disease: a randomised controlled trial. Thorax 2000;55(11):902–906.

277. Skwarska E, Cohen G, Skwarski KM, et al. Randomised controlled trial of supported discharge in patients with exacerbations of chronic obstructive pulmonary disease. Thorax 2000;55(11):907–912.

278. O'Driscoll BR, Taylor RJ, Horsley MG, Chambers DK, Bernstein A. Nebulised salbutamol with and without ipratropium bromide in acute airflow obstruction. Lancet 1989;1(8652):1418–1420.

279. Bent S, Saint S, Vittinghoff E, Grady D. Antibiotics in acute bronchitis: a meta-analysis. Am J Med 1999;107(1):62–67.

280. Saint S, Bent S, Vittinghoff E, Grady D. Antibiotics in chronic obstructive pulmonary disease exacerbations. A meta-analysis. JAMA 1995;273(12):957–960.

281. Thompson WH, Nielson CP, Carvalho P, Charan NB, Crowley JJ. Controlled trial of oral prednisone in outpatients with acute COPD exacerbation. Am J Respir Crit Care Med 1996; 154(2 Pt 1):407–412.

282. Seemungal TA, Donaldson GC, Bhowmik A, Jeffries DJ, Wedzicha JA. Time course and recovery of exacerbations in patients with chronic obstructive pulmonary disease. Am J Respir Crit Care Med 2000; 161(5):1608–1613.

283. O'Driscoll BR, Cochrane GM. Emergency use of nebulised bronchodilator drugs in British hospitals. Thorax 1987;42(7):491–493.

284. COPD Guidelines Group of the Standards of Care Committee of the BTS. BTS guidelines for the management of chronic obstructive pulmonary disease. Thorax 1997;52(Suppl 5):S1–28.

285. Niewoehner DE, Erbland ML, Deupree RH, et al. Effect of systemic glucocorticoids on exacerbations of chronic obstructive pulmonary disease. Department of Veterans Affairs Cooperative Study Group. N Engl J Med 1999;340(25):1941–1947.

286. Davies L, Angus RM, Calverley PM. Oral corticosteroids in patients admitted to hospital with exacerbations of chronic obstructive pulmonary disease: a prospective randomised controlled trial. Lancet 1999;354(9177):456–460.

Oxygen therapy and non-invasive ventilation

287. Medical Research Council Working Party. Long term domiciliary oxygen therapy in chronic hypoxic cor pulmonale complicating chronic bronchitis and emphysema. Lancet 1981;1(8222):681–686.

288. Nocturnal Oxygen Therapy Trial Group. Continuous or nocturnal oxygen therapy in hypoxemic chronic obstructive lung disease: a clinical trial. Ann Intern Med 1980; 93(3):391–398.

289. Veale D, Chailleux E, Taytard A, Cardinaud JP. Characteristics and survival of patients prescribed long-term oxygen therapy outside prescription guidelines Eur Respir J 1998;12(4):780–784.

290. Calverley PM, Leggett RJ, McElderry L, Flenley DC. Cigarette smoking and secondary polycythemia in hypoxic cor pulmonale. Am Rev Respir Dis 1982;125(5):507–510.

291. COPD Guidelines Group of the

Standards of Care Committee of the BTS. BTS guidelines for the management of chronic obstructive pulmonary disease. Thorax 1997;52(Suppl 5):S1–28.

292. Royal College of Physicians. Domiciliary oxygen therapy services. Clinical guidelines and advice for prescribers. London: Royal College of Physicians; 1999.

293. Waterhouse JC, Howard P. Breathlessness and portable oxygen in chronic obstructive airways disease. Thorax 1983;38(4):302–306.

294. Davidson AC, Leach R, George RJ, Geddes DM. Supplemental oxygen and exercise ability in chronic obstructive airways disease. Thorax 1988; 43(12):965–971.

295. Lock SH, Paul EA, Rudd RM, Wedzicha JA. Portable oxygen therapy: assessment and usage. Respir Med 1991;85(5):407–412.

296. Garrod R, Bestall JC, Paul E, Wedzicha JA. Evaluation of pulsed dose oxygen delivery during exercise in patients with severe chronic obstructive pulmonary disease. Thorax 1999;54(3):242–244.

297. Lock SH, Blower G, Prynne M, Wedzicha JA. Comparison of liquid and gaseous oxygen for domiciliary portable use. Thorax 1992; 47(2):98–100.

298. Okubadejo AA, Paul EA, Wedzicha JA. Domiciliary oxygen cylinders: indications, prescription and usage. Respir Med 1994;88(10):777–785.

299. Woodcock A, Gross ER, Geddes DM. Oxygen relieves breathlessness in 'pink puffers'. Lancet 1981;i:907–909.

300. Evans TW, Waterhouse JC, Carter A, Nicholl JF, Howard P. Short burst oxygen treatment for breathlessness in chronic obstructive airways disease. Thorax 1986;41(8):611–615.

301. Swinburn CR, Mould H, Stone TN, Corris PA, Gibson GJ. Symptomatic benefit of supplemental oxygen in hypoxemic patients with chronic lung disease. Am Rev Respir Dis 1991; 143(5 Pt 1):913–915.

302. West GA, Primeau P. Nonmedical hazards of long-term oxygen therapy. Respir Care 1983;28:906–912.

303. Elliott MW. Noninvasive ventilation in chronic obstructive pulmonary disease. N Engl J Med 1995;333(13):870–871.

304. Elliott MW. Non-invasive ventilation in chronic obstructive pulmonary disease. Br J Hosp Med 1997; 57(3):83–86.

305. Plant PK, Owen JL, Elliott MW. Early use of non-invasive ventilation for acute exacerbations of chronic obstructive pulmonary disease on general respiratory wards: a multicentre randomised controlled trial. Lancet 2000;355(9219):1931–1935.

306. Hill AT, Hopkinson RB, Stableforth DE. Ventilation in a Birmingham intensive care unit 1993–1995: outcome for patients with chronic obstructive pulmonary disease. Respir Med 1998;92:156–161.

307. Breen D, Churches T, Hawker F, Torzillo PJ. Acute respiratory failure secondary to chronic obstructive pulmonary disease treated in the intensive care unit: a long term follow up study. Thorax 2002;57(1):29–33.

308. Menzies R, Gibbons W, Goldberg P. Determinants of weaning and survival among patients with COPD who require mechanical ventilation for acute respiratory failure. Chest 1989;95:398–405.

309. Portier F, Defouilloy C, Muir JF. Determinants of immediate survival among chronic respiratory patients admitted to intensive care unit for acute respiratory failure. A prospective multicenter study. Chest 1992;101:204–210.

Pulmonary rehabilitation and non-pharmacological management

310. ATS. Pulmonary rehabilitation – 1999. Am J Respir Crit Care Med 1999;159:1666–1682.

311. Donner CF, Muir JF. Selection criteria and programmes for pulmonary rehabilitation in COPD patients. Rehabilitation and Chronic Care Scientific Group of the European Respiratory Society. Eur Respir J 1997;10(3):744–757.

312. Strijbos JH, Postma DS, van Altena R, Gimeno F, Koeter GH. A comparison between an outpatient hospital-based pulmonary rehabilitation program and a home-care pulmonary rehabilitation program in patients with COPD. A follow-up of 18 months. Chest 1996;109(2):366–372.

313. Ward JA, Akers G, Ward DG, et al. Feasibility and effectiveness of a pulmonary rehabilitation programme in a community hospital setting. Br J Gen Pract 2002;52(480):539–542.

314. Lacasse Y, Wong E, Guyatt GH, King D, Cook DJ, Goldstein RS. Meta-analysis of respiratory rehabilitation in chronic obstructive pulmonary disease. Lancet 1996;348(9035):1115–1119.

315. Pulmonary rehabilitation: joint ACCP/AACVPR evidence-based guidelines. ACCP/AACVPR Pulmonary Rehabilitation Guidelines Panel. American College of Chest Physicians. American Association of Cardiovascular and Pulmonary Rehabilitation Chest 1997; 112(5):1363–1396.

316. Schols AM, Wouters EF. Nutritional abnormalities and supplementation in chronic obstructive pulmonary disease. Clin Chest Med 2000;21(4):753–762.

317. Agusti AG. Systemic effects of chronic obstructive pulmonary disease. Novartis Found Symp 2001; 234:242–249; discussion 250–254.

318. Schols AM, Slangen J, Volovics L, Wouters EF. Weight loss is a reversible factor in the prognosis of chronic obstructive pulmonary disease. Am J Respir Crit Care Med 1998; 157(6 Pt 1):1791–1797.

319. Nichol KL, Baken L, Wuorenma J, Nelson A. The health and economic benefits associated with pneumococcal vaccination of elderly persons with chronic lung disease. Arch Intern Med 1999;159(20):2437–2442.

320. Hak E, van Essen GA, Buskens E, Stalman W, de Melker RA. Is immunising all patients with chronic lung disease in the community against influenza cost effective? Evidence from a general practice based clinical prospective cohort study in Utrecht, The Netherlands. J Epidemiol Community Health 1998;52(2):120–125.

321. Gorse GJ, Otto EE, Daughaday CC, et al. Influenza virus vaccination of patients with chronic lung disease. Chest 1997;112(5):1221–1233.

322. Chief Medical Officer. Influenza immunisation programme 2001/2002. PL/CMO/2001/4. London: Department of Health; 2001.

323. Bridges CB, Fukuda K, Cox NJ, Singleton JA. Prevention and control of influenza. Recommendations of the Advisory Committee on Immunization Practices (ACIP). MMWR Morb Mortal Wkly Rep 2001;50(RR–4):1–44.

324. Franzen D. Clinical efficacy of pneumococcal vaccination – a prospective study in patients with longstanding emphysema and/or bronchitis. Eur J Med Res 2000;5(12):537–540.

325. Prevention of pneumococcal disease: recommendations of the Advisory Committee on Immunization Practices (ACIP). MMWR Morb Mortal Wkly Rep 1997;46(RR–8):1–24.

326. Stoller JK, Hoisington E, Auger G. A

comparative analysis of arranging in-flight oxygen aboard commercial air carriers. Chest 1999;115(4):991–995.

327. Managing passengers with respiratory disease planning air travel: British Thoracic Society recommendations. Thorax 2002;57(4):289–304.

Surgical management of COPD

328. Gaensler E, Cugell D, Knudson R, et al. Surgical management of emphysema. Clin Chest Med 1983;4:443–463.

329. Pride NB, Barter CE, Hugh-Jones P. The ventilation of bullae and the effect of their removal on thoracic gas volumes and tests of over-all pulmonary function. Am Rev Respir Dis 1973;107(1):83–98.

330. Connolly JE. Results of bullectomy. Chest Surg Clin N Am 1995; 5(4):765–776.

331. Goldstraw P, Petrou M. The surgical treatment of emphysema. The Brompton approach. Chest Surg Clin N Am 1995;5(4):777–796.

332. Cooper JD, Lefrak SS. Lung-reduction surgery: 5 years on. Lancet 1999;353(suppl 1):26–27.

333. Geddes DM, Davies M, Koyama H, et al. Effect of lung-volume-reduction surgery in patients with severe emphysema. N Engl J Med 2000;343:239–245.

334. Hosenpud JD, Bennett B, Keck B, et al. The registry of the international society for heart and lung transplantation: fourteenth official report – 1997. J Heart Lung Transplant 1997;16:691–712.

335. American Thoracic Society. International guidelines for the selection of lung transplant candidates. Am J Respir Crit Care Med 1998;158:335–339.

336. Sundaresan RS, Shiraishi Y, Trulock EP, et al. Single or bilateral lung transplantation for emphysema? J Thorac Cardiovasc Surg 1996; 112(6):1485–1494; discussion 1494–1495.

337. Meyers BF, Lynch J, Trulock E, Guthrie TJ, Cooper JD, Patterson AG. Lung transplantation: a decade of experience. Ann Surg 1999;230(3):362–371.

338. Corris PA. Lung transplantation for chronic obstructive pulmonary disease: an exercise in quality rather than quantity? Thorax 1999; 54(Suppl 2):S24–S27.

New treatments

339. Barnes PJ. Novel approaches and targets for treatment of chronic obstructive pulmonary disease. Am J Respir Crit Care Med 1999;160(5 Pt 2):S72–S79.

340. Goswami SK, Kivity S, Marom Z. Erythromycin inhibits respiratory glycoconjugate secretion from human airways in vitro. Am Rev Respir Dis 1990;141(1):72–78.

341. Johnson DC. A role for phosphodiesterase type-4 inhibitors in COPD? Lancet 2001; 358(9278):256–257.

Palliative care

342. Gore JM, Brophy CJ, Greenstone MA. How well do we care for patients with end stage chronic obstructive pulmonary disease (COPD)? A comparison of palliative care and quality of life in COPD and lung cancer. Thorax 2000; 55(12):1000–1006.

343. Sullivan KE, Hebert PC, Logan J, O'Connor AM, McNeely PD. What do physicians tell patients with end-stage COPD about intubation and mechanical ventilation? Chest 1996;109(1):258–264.

344. Skilbeck J, Mott L, Page H, Smith D, Hjelmeland-Ahmedzai S, Clark D. Palliative care in chronic obstructive airways disease: a needs assessment. Palliat Med 1998;12:245–254.

345. Corner J, Plant H, A'Hern R, Bailey C.

Non-pharmacological intervention for breathlessness in lung cancer. Palliat Med 1996;10:299–305.

346. Garner S, Eldridge F, Wagner PG, Dowell RT. Buspirone, an anxiolytic drug that stimulates respiration. Am Rev Respir Dis 1989;139:946–950.

347. British Medical Association. Advance statements about medical treatment. London: British Medical Association; 1995.

348. Curtis JR, Wenrich MD, Carline JD, Shannon SE, Ambrozy DM, Ramsey PG. Patients' perspectives on physician skill in end-of-life care: differences between patients with COPD, cancer, and AIDS. Chest 2002;122(1):356–362.

Practice organization

349. Watson PB, Town GI, Holbrook N, Dwan C, Toop LJ, Drennan CJ. Evaluation of a self-management plan for chronic obstructive pulmonary disease. Eur Respir J 1997; 10(6):1267–1271.

350. Stothard A, Brewer K. Dramatic improvement in COPD patient care in nurse-led clinic. Nurs Times 2001; 97(24):36–37.

351. Whatling J. The role of the nurse in the management of COPD and asthma. Prim Care Respir J 2001;10(4):95–96.

352. Gallefoss F, Bakke PS. Impact of patient education and self-management on morbidity in asthmatics and patients with chronic obstructive pulmonary disease. Respir Med 2000;94(3):279–287.

353. Emery CF, Schein RL, Hauck ER, MacIntyre NR. Psychological and cognitive outcomes of a randomized trial of exercise among patients with chronic obstructive pulmonary disease. Health Psychol 1998;17(3):232–240.

354. Pulmonary rehabilitation. Thorax 2001;56(11):827–834.

355. Gallefoss F, Bakke PS, Kjaersgaard P. Quality of life assessment after patient education in a randomized controlled study on asthma and chronic obstructive pulmonary disease. Am J Respir Crit Care Med 1999; 159(3):812–817.

356. Littlejohns P, Baveystock CM, Parnell H, Jones PW. Randomised controlled trial of the effectiveness of a respiratory health worker in reducing impairment, disability, and handicap due to chronic airflow limitation. Thorax 1991; 46(8):559–564.

357. Cockcroft A, Bagnall P, Heslop A, et al. Controlled trial of respiratory health worker visiting patients with chronic respiratory disability. BMJ (Clin Res Ed) 1987;294(6566):225–228.

358. Bergner M, Hudson LD, Conrad DA, et al. The cost and efficacy of home care for patients with chronic lung disease. Med Care 1988;26(6):566–579.

359. Smith BJ, Appleton SL, Bennett PW, et al. The effect of a respiratory home nurse intervention in patients with chronic obstructive pulmonary disease (COPD). Aust N Z J Med 1999; 29(5):718–725.

360. Smith B, Appleton S, Adams R, Southcott A, Ruffin R. Home care by outreach nursing for chronic obstructive pulmonary disease (Cochrane Review). In: The Cochrane Library. Oxford: Update Software; 2002.

LIST OF PATIENT QUESTIONS

INDEX

*Numbers in **bold** refer to figures, tables and boxes*